LADY OF GRAY
HEALING CANDIDA
THE
NIGHTMARE CHEMICAL EPIDEMIC

by Elizabeth Rose

THIRD EDITION

BUTTERFLY PUBLISHING COMPANY
2210 WILSHIRE BLVD.
SUITE 845
SANTA MONICA, CALIF. 90403
(213) 829-2002

Library of Congress catalog card number 85-070122
ISBN 0-9614637-0-8

1. The Twelve Steps reprinted for adaption with permission of Alcoholics Anonymous World Services Inc:

1. We admitted we were powerless over alcohol - that our lives had become unmanageable.
2. Came to believe that a Power greater than ourselves could restore us to sanity.
3. Made a decision to turn our will and our lives over to the care of God as we understood him.
4. Made a searching and fearless moral inventory of ourselves.
5. Admitted to God, to ourselves, and to another human being the exact nature of our wrongs.
6. Were entirely ready to have God remove all these defects of character.
7. Humbly asked Him to remove our shortcomings.
8. Made a list of all persons we had harmed, and became willing to make amends to them all.
9. Made direct amends to such people wherever possible, except when to do so would injure them or others.
10. Continued to take personal inventory and when we were wrong promptly admitted it.
11. Sought through prayer and meditation to improve our conscious contact with God as we understood Him, praying only for knowledge of His will and the power to carry that out.
12. Having had a spiritual awakening as the result of these steps, we try to carry this message to alcoholics, and to practice these principles in all our affairs.

1. We admitted we were powerless over chemicals — that our life had become unmanageable.
2. Came to believe that a Power greater than ourselves could restore us to sanity from the brain toxicity.
3. Made a decision to turn our will and our lives over to the care of God, *as we understood Him.*
4. Made a searching and fearless moral inventory of ourselves.
4. Admitted to ourselves, and to another human being the nature of our faults, then surrendering them to a Higher Power.
6. From this inventory, made a list of our character defects.
7. Humbly ask our Higher Power to remove these defects of character.
8. Made a list of people to whom we owed amends.
9. Made amends without bringing harm to ourselves or *anyone* else.
10. Took a daily inventory of assets and liabilities to keep ourselves balanced, immediately forgiving ourselves for wrong actions, and asking assistance to strengthen us while crediting ourselves for loving actions.
11. Sought through prayer and meditation a conscious contact with God.
12. Having had a spiritual awakening as a result of these steps, we tried to carry the message to other candidiasis sufferers, and to practice these principles in all our affairs.

2. The KIVA Process experimental information printed by permission of Orie Bachechi, owner KIVA Incorporated.

ISBN 0-9614637-1-6

CONTENTS

PREFACE

This book was written to give hope to the critically ill person with E.I. and systemic candidiasis. As a result of my personal Gethsemane, many blessings have entered my life. I look forward to sharing with you how it was for me and how it became.

This is a book about love — love for the seriously ill people with systemic Candidiasis, my fellow sufferers of this man-made 20th Century malady. Without the need to help allay your suffering through sharing my experience, strength, and hope, this book would not have been written.

Doctors, biochemists, researchers and physicists are presently working overtime trying to find answers to this Apocalypse. Many of them know of my story and telephone me to give hope and inspiration to the suffering souls behind me. Since I was *the* most critically ill case the doctors had seen to date in October of 1981 (they dared not touch me, for I went into allergic shock [anaphylaxis] from food, air, water and clothing — death is the usual prognosis), my comeback was even all the more phenomenal.

I am greatly indebted to Eve Bergman, who taught me much of what healed me physically, to Dr. Stig Erlander, a biochemist, whom I credit with saving my life at the nadir of the illness, to Dr. Steven Levine, a biochemist, and fellow sufferer who gave me hope when there was none, to Zena Malek, my psychotherapist, who pulled me through many hours of suicidal reactions, to Tom Carmichael, who gave me hugs and compassion when I needed it most, to Brenda Almeda, a sufferer of another immune disease, who shared my agony with humor, to Dr. Luc D'Ardenness, a physician and friend, who contributed to this book and to my recovery, to Jen and Amy, my daughters who loved me through all of this, but especially to God, who healed me.

FOREWORD

No one among us likes to believe we have created a man-made chemical horror producing previously unknown immune diseases that presently permeate the planet. Epidemics—AIDS, ARCS [AIDS related complex], the silent chemical epidemic, systemic Candidiasis which develops into the deadly Environmental Illness [80 million plus cases estimated in the U.S. alone], Epstein-Barr, Multiple Sclerosis, Lupus, bizarre cancers and other immunity malfunctions, will be the door for millions to the Golden Life of Englightenment that has already begun for many.

How do I know? Systemic yeast or *Candida Albicans,* in an AIDS-like effect, completely shattered my immune system, a direct result of acute chemical poisoning, leaving me critically ill and physically isolated for seven years, during which I had *two* near-death experiences and hovered at the edge of death on approximately fifty other occasions. During this terror filled time, my being opened up to information unknown to scientists or anyone else—and me an atheist—to help the planet with the many immune problems assaulting the people. We cannot survive in the 20th Century without our immunity to toxic chemicals. This living-death, known by the innocuous name "Environmental Illness", results from the immune system being exposed to severe stresses, either singularly or to combined physical, mental, emotional and spiritual ones, thereby causing an overgrowth of the benign fungus, *Candida,* which spreads throughout the body, bringing about a very slow, nightmarish death. AIDS and ARCS victims usually die from the complications of *Candida.* The significance in our lives today of all these yeast-related maladies was guided to me while in a meditative state and confirmed by direct guidance to several places in the Bible.

Corinthians 5:6-7—"Do you not know that a little yeast has its effect through the dough? Get rid of the old yeast to make of yourselves fresh dough . . . Let us celebrate the feast [Passover] not with the old yeast, but with the unleavened bread of sincerity and truth," *St. Paul the Apostle.* This particular statement addresses moral bankruptcy and the need to purify it from one's system in order for the new "dough"—The New Self—to emerge.

Again in Galatians 6:7, a further reference is made to losing the spiritual path of life—"You were progressing so very well; who diverted you from the path of truth? Such enticement does not come from Him who calls you. A little yeast can effect the entire dough." The "yeast" rotting the entire "loaf" is the improper use of freedom. As a planet, we must plead guilty as charged. As a result, yeast related diseases manifest themselves—and all immune breakdowns are fungus related—awakening us to the soul sickness within.

Only the asleep—more people than we realize—will journey this rugged road. The immune disease manifested in an individual will be based on four factors: genetic predisposition, personality type, environment, and soul choice. At the same time, new healing methods have entered the planet to aid the spiritual transformation of persons who chose to enter the New Life, thereby enabling them to avoid the nightmarish suffering of these awakener ailments.

Our bodies are being changed right down to the cellular level, a new atomic structure being created in which the new consciousness evolved will make the spiritual body visible to the naked eye. The year is not clear; The Way is here.

ARCS et al is really a mutated cell developed from chemical pollution of the body, including man-made vaccines containing this cellular material, that permits the immune system to be eventually destroyed. When a person pollutes "the self" with drugs, alcohol, unloving sex, chemical preservatives, vaccines, and chronic inhalation of toxic materials such as formaldehyde, pesticides, tar fumes, paint, solvents, and other petrochemical products, the body rebels. The immune system becomes depressed and damaged, allowing the overgrowth of *Candida* on the mucous membranes—nasal, oral, intestinal, vaginal, and rectal—thereby releasing seventy toxins per cell into the hosts' bodies and bloodstreams.

Mankind is not meant to live with hundreds of toxic chemicals accumulating in the tissues. And they do build up, staying in the cells for as long as 20 years *before* serious physical illness appears. Those who develop critical illnesses at young ages incarnated already polluted via their parents' toxic bodies. Anyone under the age of forty is more vulnerable to these types of breakdowns. Why? The pesticides, plastics, antibiotics and other petrochemically derived drugs manifested in the early 1940's have had *forty plus years* to work on our immune systems. Chemical prosperity misused brought with it chemical destruction of life on our planet.

Yet we mustn't despair, for the Divine Law of Physics states that each action contains an opposite and equal reaction. Therefore, despite chemical pollution of the plant being at its Zenith, the Energies of the Universe at the opposite end of this spectrum are equally here to assist us to transform and survive. The next question then is: How are we to do this?

Free energy is the source of all light. New inventions and healing methods are being produced to harness this magnificent power many of us are already feeling. The magicians of the New Life are old souls, many transformed Atlanteans in origin, who developed and misused these powers once before, thereby losing the knowledge of the Great Crystal or atomic energy [God Incarnate] employed in a non-polluting, non-controlling manner; they are back to help resolve their own karma by helping the world in its rectification.

The KIVA light, a normal looking four-foot flourescent tube—its effect is peacefulness, not the agitation one experiences around toxic yellow-white fluorescents—emanating a blue-white spectrum of color [the central core, crystal color of the earth density], activates the pineal gland, the master of the immune system, the material version of the third or "all-knowing eye", creating vast energy which enhances calcium production, the number one mineral upon which all other body minerals are dependent for genesis, the result being the body heals itself *and* generates its own vitamins, minerals, amino acids and other necessary ingredients to sustain a positive life force. A side effect of using the light is that old emotional scars regurgitate and are healed—permanently.

The "N" machine, a gyroscope with two magnets, harnesses free energy or the life force we can feel but not see so that man can utilize its cheap, non-polluting power to electrate the home and run the car, factories and office buildings. The U.S. government recently granted the first patent for this Teslaarchetype machine after decades of exhaustive fighting by the enlightened physicists-inventors.

However, the greatest "Machine" coming to us at this time is the "New-Life" body, a crystal-created universe center from which will emanate seemingly magical powers. Although this transition of this "new body" will be a difficult one, it can be alleviated by people's conscious, *collective* efforts to change via communal cooperation.

The primary way an individual can help create the New Body is through one's *own* transformation: This means going through and transcending our physical, emotional, and mental limits to a higher state of consciousness in which all is Light.

How do we do this? By educating ourselves as to how we are polluting our own minds and bodies on a daily basis, and *consciously* committing ourselves to beginning a gradual change. It isn't easy, but necessary if we are to avoid the toxic states I have described. Are you eating contaminated food and drinking sick water? If you are, you are making yourself very vulnerable to the life-threatening degenerative diseases.

Begin by cleaning up your environment within and without. A slow process at best, but nevertheless a beginning—that is all that is needed. Do *something! Anything!* That's how transformation occurs—step by baby step. Use the KIVA light to detoxify your home and water, being sure to have glass bottled water only as plastic is toxic and leeches into the water.

Once you've begun purifying your environment, begin purifying your mind. The KIVA Light releases trapped emotions registered as lesions or scars on the central nervous system while simultaneously healing the body's physical damage and regenerating the central nervous system cell by cell. When the growth appears too rapid for your constitution, turn off the light and the healing process immediately halts. *You are in full charge of your transformation.*

The emotions must also be healed. Two new ways have entered our knowledge. The super-consciousness tapes channeled through me while critically ill harness the new energies blasting the earth at this present time. They bring about instant healing and transformation at the cellular level. These higher energy tapes work passively through energy fields for those too ill—or too lazy—to do the work, creating an expanding spiritual body manifested as heat or warmth surrounding the body.

The second instant healer revealed is the use of healing anything by channeling flower energy of the etheric feminine creative force. The simplest way to do this is to envision your favorite flower for that day and "eat" it spiritually, then surrounding the physical body and chakras with the etheric essence. There are more advanced techniques but you have to be ready for them, and you already have a lot of work to do: I've shown you a starter method.

The healing must be instant now for the time grows short for mankind to awaken to what it has done to itself. New ways of transforming to the New Self will be the salvation of the planet. Madame Blavatsky's pioneer work with light streams has been expanded to encompass *how* to use them along with etheric flower energies, chakras, Hierarchal Zodiac Overlords, and the new energy manifesting from Ragna or the twelfth Buddhic plane which had not manifested physically before in this eternity system. Through this new information, these who are ready will be transformed to "beings of light" or great crystals. The Christ or Cosmic Consciousness will appear in a physical form when the Christ manifests in the majority of the earth souls' hearts. The best way to bring this about is to *heal yourself.*

Fear not the antichrist-antechrist energies for the master teachers are reversing and transforming their power. The time has come for us to benefit from and live Jesus's words: "As I do, so ye shall do greater. . ." It is promised. He just didn't say when: it is *now* as evidenced by the appearance of the quasi-Supernova on February 23 of 1987, manifesting between the veils of the outgoing Piscean age and the incoming Aquarian: The brilliant star is the formation from energy of the Second Coming Christ Light.

The souls most prone to the chemical breakdown of the immune system are the allergic, obsessive-compulsives whose bodies are more sensitive then the ordinary person; they are also more prone to drug and alcohol addiction.

The homosexual population contains large numbers of these types of individuals. Many abuse substances and themselves to an extreme; they have not been singled out, for a great deal of the rest of the population does the exact same thing. Therefore, homosexuals are not being punished as many believe, but are old souls whose high creativity level and ability to generate money will work hardest to find answers to AIDS, a blessing disguised as a bringer of great pain.

The opportunity presents itself to utilize one's hidden powers to bring solutions to earth's dilemma. Fear not because your path is life-threatening disease—you are an example of the New Life, the transformation in progress.

Hence we must look at all these horror immune diseases as an opening to join in the transformation to the New Life or, leave the planet. It is that simple. That's what this book intends to teach.

—Blessings and Health,
Elizabeth Rose

PART I

THE STORY

THE BREAKDOWN

Carrying seriously ill nine-month old baby . . . Huge pin-wheel shaped kaleidoscope eyes . . . Dizzy, spinning, brain whirling . . . Go to doctor's office . . . Sit baby on desk . . . Doctor and I discuss her case . . . She picks up a bottle of phenobarb and eats it . . . I can't take my eyes off this baby for one second or disaster strikes . . . Baby loses consciousness . . . Rush "it" to hospital . . . Emergency Room . . . Falls off stretcher while I'm not looking . . . Now I'm Head Nurse . . . Must decide . . . Lavage overdose first or check head injury . . . Rush to operating room . . . See myself bent, broken by disease . . . Want to be rid of this baby . . . Despairing about survival . . . Toxic poisoning . . . . . . How much longer could I bear the burden of this nightmarish illness? Still alive . . . In my bedroom . . . In Berkeley . . . .

What a terrifying dream! *Thank God, I'm awake now.* I lie in my attic bedroom, alone, shivering with fear. Although the scene was only a dream, one fact was perfectly clear — in the *real* world, I knew I was dying.

How had this happened to me, I asked my ashen body? How has a healthy, sexy, tall, vital woman in her thirties become, almost overnight, a victim of the 20th Century's most pervasive horror of an epidemic to befall mankind since bubonic plague in the Middle Ages — the man-made disease, systemic Candidiasis.

How was I to know those early symptoms would lead to this? My mind races back to the summer of '76, when I was biking with my friend Michael, a mathematician, along the Manhattan Beach bicycle path. Southern California was having one of her usual smoggy days — a fact I'd long ago accustomed myself to. Suddenly I experienced severe chest pain on the right side of my breastbone. Inhaling was extremely difficult as if someone had built a cement wall inside my lung. My friend helped me back to his house. Nothing serious, I thought, probably induced by smog.

The pain continued. Pale and shaken, stubbornly I drove myself home. As the day wore on the pain increased. By evening, I could not lie down as the pain increased one hundred-fold, and I had great difficulty breathing. My husband took me to an internist friend. ''Pulmonary embolus,'' he declared seriously. *My God, can't be — a person drops dead instantly from that condition unattended!* I should know. My profession had been nursing, specialty emergency room. I'd seen instant death from a blood clot in the lung. The doctor wanted to hospitalize me, but very frightened and still obstinate, I felt safer at home and agreed to be admitted in the morning. This day was the beginning of a six-year descent into hell.

In the morning, a CAT scan showed a quarter-sized marking on my right lung. Terror struck my gut. Yet something wasn't right, for despite running IV heparin (an anticoagulant) the pain continued. Three days later, the pain subsided and the doctor released me that weekend. This ended my first episode. Incidentally, I was a smoker who kept right on smoking. No one seemed to notice the importance of this habit.

My deteriorating marriage had reached its final destination. Shortly afterwards I left my husband and spent a week of summer in Lake Tahoe. Breathing was labored at this high altitude. Frightening. A subsequent trip in August to Hawaii to visit a recently divorced woman friend, with my daughters Amy age 4 and Jen (short for Jennifer) age 7, proved to be the culmination of my nightmare. Exhaustion was the common symptom accompanying me now most of the time. I could barely stand up at all. Out of nowhere my body took on the consistency of lead. As I debarked the plane, the sweltering Hawaiian humidity hit me in the face like a wall of steam. I couldn't breathe. My color turned gray and I began gasping for air. Panic seized my heart. Ninety-eight humidity, 98° — a killer. My girlfriend Jeannie, divorced mother of four children under the age of 8, picked us up. She noticed my color and asked, very concerned, what was wrong with me. ''I don't know,'' came my shaky reply. Fortunately for me, she resided in Kihei on Maui — the desert region of the island. Although the daily wind was akin to Santa Anas, I felt better when we arrived in this region. This was a vacation? I checked in with a local doctor for weekly blood tests. I asked him if I had hypoglycemia. His method of checking was to give me a spoonful of sugar and observe me for twenty minutes. To begin with I argued with him that this test was not accurate and sugar would make me worse. But this was in the days when I still allowed the doctor to be the ''expert'' on my body.

At first I became high, then suddenly, I felt irritable, angry, agitated and faint. He poo-pooed my reaction and said it wasn't hypoglycemia, just ''anxiety.'' My deep inner rage was beginning to build up at doctors like him. As I left his office I asked him to explain my color — gray. He said he couldn't. A wasted journey to Lahaina, the other side of the island.

I stumbled along this way, unable to sleep at night because I couldn't inhale properly. Fear was growing in my mind — *What was wrong with me that clinical tests didn't show?* At this point, I decided to reserve a room at the Intercontinental Hotel. Just walking into the air-conditioned room relieved my symptoms.

Newly separated from my husband, I decided to go dancing and have some fun in the hotel ballroom with my girlfriend Jeannie. I met a lovely, blue-eyed, blond-haired Italian from Rome, who was training at Cornell University in hotel management. Unbeknownst to me, my acquaintance with Roberto was very fortunate for me that night — for I didn't know what was coming.

While dancing a very strenuous number, severe chest pain grabbed my entire lungs. Doubling over, clutching my dress and hiding my alarm, I asked my new friend to help me to my room. My girls were sleeping and I let the babysitter go, acting as if nothing were wrong. Only a strong mind could survive the terrifying symptoms I'm about to describe, for this was merely the beginning of my hell.

Unexpectedly I became high as a kite, then everything started going black. Terrified of losing control and passing out, I fought to stay conscious. *What in God's name was happening to me?* Roberto took total charge, calling an ambulance and hotel management to send a person to stay with the children. He stayed behind with my girls to explain my disappearance, while I was sped through the roads of Maui to the only hospital. My mind raced in my semi-conscious state — *Oh Lord, please, don't let me be seriously ill in a foreign port where I know no one.* (Unfortunately, my girlfriend thought I'd found ''instant romance'' and never checked to see where I was.) In the emergency room, a strange doctor greeted me, the partner of my original physician who was off that night. Looking out through a gray fog, I felt only one emotion — sheer terror. My old nursing head appeared. I wanted to be running this drama, not the cause of it. With my history of pulmonary embolus, the physician placed me in the Intensive Care Unit.

The next few hours are very vague. In and out of consciousness. Severe chest pain. I'd had a few drinks that evening which frightened me from taking any medication at all, for I'd been so drug-sensitive all my life. By 4:00AM, the pain was totally unbearable, so I requested Demerol. The rest is very foggy but I seem to recall abruptly ''going out.'' The next thing I knew, I was on the ceiling looking down on my very gray body sitting upright in the hospital bed. Doctors and nurses were hovering around; tubes and equipment were everywhere. Then all went blank. Around 7:00AM I awakened and asked the nurse what happened. She said, ''After the shot, we almost lost you last night.''

Later on that week when I was out of danger, a second lung scan was performed. The results showed multiple black spots all over both lungs. The doctors were extremely concerned, yet puzzled too, for lungs full of emboli are fatal. And I was alive. Fear became my constant companion. To deal with all this terror, I had Jeannie sneak bottles of beer into my room and we'd laugh and drink together. Being an ex-nurse, I knew all the hospital tricks and planned our drinks between temperatures and blood tests. A crazy way to deal with the situation, but the best I could do under the circumstances.

Three weeks later, the doctors released me, with great trepidation, to fly solo five hours back to Los Angeles with my two children. They'd placed me on massive doses of coumadin, an anti-coagulant, whereby a skin nick could prove fatal through bleeding to death.

Jeannie took me to the airport. Upon hitting the Hawaiian air, I turned gray again, gasping for air. So determined am I, that I insisted on flying home anyway. Once more, my body was leaden. Yet right after the air-conditioning was started in the plane I felt a lot better. Waves of unconsciousness came and went during the flight. Keep calm, this will pass, my numb mind repeated over and over.

My brother John and his wife Barbara picked me up in a wheelchair at the airport. I broke into tears at seeing human faces I knew who cherished and loved me. They sped me to San Pedro Hospital's emergency room. I began to lose consciousness again. They called in a cardiovascular specialist. After an arterial blood gas, he still couldn't figure out what was wrong. Still, he told me it wasn't serious. I knew his tests had their limits and I had to fight for my life now. I asked my brother to sign me out. He did. At this point, I was fearful of dying and enraged at being told, one more time, "it" was "anxiety." I was determined to find my own answer.

Back in my own house, the condition subsided for a few days. On top of all this trauma, severe lower back pain developed with intermittent numbness in both legs.

Two surgeons declared I needed immediate surgery. A divorce, lung disease and back surgery simultaneously — enough stress to kill a person. At the same time, my mother surrogate died in September and my father-in-law in October. Blanking out the pain with alcohol and not thinking, focusing straight ahead on what had to be done, was how I survived. My maternal grandmother had an anesthesia death, so I informed my doctors that I was lung impaired and highly allergic. They listened and had a super-specialist anesthesiologist on my case.

The surgery was delayed five months while I found someone to come live-in and care for my two children and myself. My almost ex-husband disappeared in every way but financially. Although I didn't believe in God, some intuition told me to turn everything over to Him — the surgeon, the surgery and my fear. This calmed my mind and made life easier.

A four-hour laminectomy was performed in March of '77. The pain was relieved. The surgeon discovered the 4th lumbar vertebrae turned over almost parallel to the others. During my stay at the hospital, a female friend brought me a small bottle of wine. Somehow, pumped full of post-operative drugs, I drank the entire bottle of wine and blacked out. The nurses told me the next day, I climbed out of bed and was discovered in a hall closet. When they placed me back in bed, I cried for hours over the demise of my marriage. I remembered absolutely nothing.

Prior to the surgery I'd been placed on all kinds of narcotics. Percodan caused my worst reaction. Nausea and vomiting occurred, then "verbal diarrhea" and blackouts (Friends told me months later I called on the phone from 11PM to 4AM. One friend bathed, fed and put her baby to bed while I spoke. Another put the phone by his ear and went to sleep. I remembered nothing.) The usual treatment after back surgery is Valium to allay the severe leg cramps. I became severely depressed on it and threw them out. The bitter divorce continued.

All went well physically for about two months. Pain-free, I built up my strength by walking up and down my large home daily. The doctor ordered physical therapy. From the lengthy twisting of my spine to the left side I'd developed strictures in my right hip. When they went to bend my right leg I screamed with pain. This was a setback. My surgeon who was very upset by this even ordered me to bed for two more months. This caved me in emotionally — I could not bear that on top of everything else. I had planned to be well — this demoralized me. If I couldn't walk and care for myself I felt worthless and would surely go mad; I began to drink too much. In less than a month I gained 30 pounds. My body became bloated and I could press my skin in anywhere and it would stay that way. I knew I was toxic but didn't know what to do.

The severe stress of my divorce went on and on. It was all I could do to survive that emotionally without the added stress of being physically crippled. I could not stand or sit for more than twenty minutes before I had to lie down. I felt as if my back were broken. Ironically, it *was* in many ways.

By June of '78, I knew I was really ill but still couldn't find an answer. I went from doctor to doctor, unsuccessfully. Paramedics rescued me on three occasions as I blacked out in restaurants. "Anxiety" over my divorce was the consensus. "Malarkey" I said — I'm a strong, independent individual and something was drastically wrong with me.

One morning I drank some instant decaffinated coffee. Five minutes later I felt stoned out of my head. All went gray in front of my eyes, and I fell to the floor. Terrified, I crawled to the phone and called my next-door neighbor and friend Dr. Marx, a gynecologist. Almost completely paralyzed! Speech slurred. Saliva drooled from my mouth. He rushed over and said "God, Elizabeth, I don't know what's wrong with you — try some orange juice. It might be hypoglycemia." By the way, I was still on the floor when he arrived, unable to get up. The paralysis lessened. I crawled up to the couch badly shaken and begged him not to leave me alone. Tears streamed down my face. He stayed until the episode spontaneously subsided.

There is a factor I've forgotten to mention, a clue to the mosaic being formed by my disease.

In 1970, I started using a two-process dyeing system to color my chestnut brown hair almost platinum blonde. Within a year, my head began burning upon each application. Right after my second daughter Amy was born in 1972, I had a serious reaction to hair dye in the beauty parlor — hives, blisters on my scalp, shaking chills, wax-colored skin, pulse and heartbeat at least 140, feeling of dying — a fading that begins in one's extremities. You feel the life force leaving your body. Even in shock I was so stubborn and perfectionistic, I refused to have an ambulance called. I knew this was anaphylaxis — an acute allergic reaction. Luckily, I didn't die.

After the reaction subsided spontaneously, I rushed to a dermatologist's office. Dr. White concluded I was allergic to hair dye and told me to stop using it. I stopped using it — for a year. Willfully, I returned to brown dye to cover my few gray strands. Mentioning these facts is very important and will prove the key to the diagnosis of my ailment. Little did I know, all the time, hair dye was the major factor beginning my physical breakdown.

COMPLETE EXHAUSTION

The next phase of the breakdown was complete exhaustion. Total debilitation after the back surgery on an occasional basis. By 1979, the exhaustion was almost as constant as was the craving for alcohol. Unable to function without it, I realized, sickeningly, I was addicted. It was the only relief I got from the exhaustion. I entered Alcoholics Anonymous in June of '79 — dying — with continuous toxic brain symptoms — paranoia, peripheral hallucinations, fear, agitation, depression and extreme negative thinking. I thought alcohol was my problem. It proved to be only one of them.

Now I craved ice cream and peanuts all the time. If I didn't eat one or the other, I became shocky — sweats, faintness, very low blood pressure and pulse. Yet something new was added. Only eating *huge* amounts of ice cream — ½ gallon — stopped these cravings. Moments later, my extremities were a blue-purple, my body the color of a cadaver. I'd become mentally confused and begin to lose consciousness. Forcing myself to vomit stopped the symptoms. Fear was my constant, black companion now. Massive amounts of peanuts also stopped the cravings but, strangely enough, I kept losing weight. I dropped 20 pounds in two weeks in September of '79, for which I was deeply grateful for I'd not enjoyed being fat. Continuous obsessive thinking had become my personality. I was not this way before all this happened to me, as my close friends could attest.

In July 1980 I met a man named Jean-Pierre and fell in love. He was a tall madonna-eyed Adonis from Paris. On our second date, we attended the Greek Theater after eating a scrumptuous pizza. One could smell marijuana all over the open smoggy air. Suddenly I felt weak, began sweating and saw my color was gray. Double vision ensued. I grabbed his coat sleeve, embarrassed and frightened. He was very kind and asked what he could do to help. "Hold me," I replied shaken, for I didn't *know* what to do. A cool breeze appeared and the marijuana smoke was blown away. I didn't black out, but came very close. Jean-Pierre seemed very concerned and wanted to know if doctors could help me. I replied, ''No — no one knows what is wrong with me.'' He was very compassionate — I decided to keep him around.

Trying to have a love affair in this condition is like falling in love and dating while in a bed in the Intensive Care Unit. Fortunately, I'd met a kind and understanding human being who didn't think this was all in my head. This gave me great comfort as nothing much else did those days.

By January of '81, further deterioration set in. I had progressed to either going insane out of nowhere or sliding into unconsciousness as if I'd been given general anesthesia in the smoky AA meetings. I continued to share my terror at meetings — some thought I was insane, others had compassion for me. Rages appeared from nowhere totally unrelated to reality. *This is it — I'm surely going mad just like my father.* He'd died of cancer of the bone marrow, plus alcoholism. I was progressing similarly to him, with the exception that he developed cancer whereas my ailment mystified all.

A brand new symptom developed at this time. A flu-like syndrome began on a daily basis. Simultaneously, ice cream cravings increased. If I didn't eat the ''fix,'' I had violent shaking and ''madness'' in my head. On the contrary, if I did eat the ice cream, I became weak, faint, severely nauseated and vomited. Either way, I couldn't win. I had this whole secret life going on, ashamed of my lack of control over my food cravings. Although I'd been off alcohol 15 months, my health was deteriorating. My AA friends had no answers. Funny — after I ate dairy of any kind I'd awaken the next day with my eyeballs feeling like ground glass, my legs numb and weak, and pressure on my chest as if the cosmos were sitting on it. (Once the disease reaches this stage it progresses rapidly).

A continuous fear of ''cracking'' alternating with depression was added on in February of '81. Anger, uncontrollable anger, was my alter ego. Interspersed with all this suffering was my back — unhealed from surgery — dislocating at the slightest move, crippling me and placing me in excruciating pain. There were many days I wanted to die. I'd relied on my independent nature all my life and it had served me well. But for reasons yet unknown to me, I was brought to my knees with suffering and a strong sense of powerlessness. I felt lost on top of my brain increasingly being fogged and spacey, leaving me unable to think or function on an intellectual level. Neither could I add or subtract, nor barely read anymore. Surely, I convinced myself, this was the irreversible brain damage of alcoholism. But I didn't drink long enough for that to happen.

An intimate relationship became progressively impossible for I began to collapse and be semi-conscious. The terror was increasing. Personal problems were piling on top of my head. The stress I was under should have killed me — it didn't. For I was in the the throes of a living death.

I'd given up on doctors by now. Conversely, my visit to my daughter Amy's pediatrician proved to be a turning point providing me with a key to my dilemma. This was July 9, 1981. Amy's doctor suspected she had allergies and recommended a workup by a Dr. Lisot. A very personable man, he explained Amy had classic tree and weed allergies and needed treatment. A light went on in my head. *Suppose I'm allergic? Could that be it?* So I signed up for the same tests.

When I told him my history of drug allergies, naming names like a pharmacopedia, Dr. Lisot looked at me suspiciously. I laughed.

''Dr. Lisot, I'm an R.N., I know drugs inside out.'' That misunderstanding resolved, we proceeded with the tests. Lo and behold, I was allergic to all milk, cheese, grains, peanuts, walnuts and some fruits, especially citrus — about thirty foods in all. This was very depressing. As low as I felt, I eliminated most of these foods immediately. I dropped ten pounds in two weeks. Slim and svelte again, it was one consolation in this nightmare.

You think this solved my problem? Oh no — I began reacting worse to brown dye and shampoo. Hives around my forehead, burning, and redness on my scalp. I went for a body wave and had chemical burns on my neck, turned gray and had shaking chills. Began losing consciousness. The owner was shook. I'd asked Lisot previously if this procedure was safe for me. He said it was. I stumbled to the pay phone in the beauty parlor and called him. ''You have anaphylaxis,'' he said, ''and hydrocardon allergy.'' He told me to come right over. Patiently and sympathetically, he explained first, my anaphylaxis, on a scale of one to ten, was a nine. (Anaphylaxis is an allergic reaction to a substance which leads to collapse and death — a classic example is a person receiving a pencillin injection and dying five minutes later.) It was a shock to find not only was I seriously ill, but I must avoid all hydrocarbons. When he told me the list I almost fainted. Shampoo, soap, detergent, cosmetics, creams, carpets, paint, rugs, furniture, synthetic clothing, walls, floors, cars and on and on. This covered everything we live with. Little did I digest at that time how serious this was, for my emotional shock protected me.

Meanwhile, my relationship with Jean-Pierre became stormy. Discovering he had lied to me about being divorced six weeks into the relationship surely didn't help my medical condition. Out of nowhere, he phoned to tell me he was only separated for two years, not divorced. The wife and children living at the other end of the state made the lie an easy one for him. Rage churned inside me towards him. So overwhelmed was I at this point with the stress in my own life and not wanting one more drop, I told him to get a divorce or get out of my life.

Reluctantly, he filed, about a month later. My heart told me this man was going nowhere and neither were we; my emotions said, ''Hang on to his love, flawed as this relationship is — you need him.'' And so I did. In California, divorce is final in six months. He filed in October of '80 — he'd be free in April of '81. The severe stress I was under being so ill clouded my perceptions. I decided not to make any decisions concerning him, *no matter what*. My health was so fragile, the stress of breaking up would have been very detrimental.

In January, Jean-Pierre lost a bundle in the stock market, leaving him emotionally paralyzed. He also kept coming up with excuses for prolonging the divorce. April came and went. I was enraged at his weakness but continued to see him, berating myself daily for being weak and needing him. All these factors added more apples to an already full barrel. It was only a matter of time before the barrel ruptured.

By June 1981, gray most days, my brain totally fogged, and unable to stand up, my life became narrower and narrower. Jean-Pierre laughed, trying to make light of my condition when I called him at work, semi-conscious, slurring, ''I'm drunk without drinking, and can't get off my bed.''

Fortunately for me, I met a fellow sufferer named Karen. We called each other daily, discussing L.A.'s air. We believed it was the entire problem. The summer of '81 was the smoggiest L.A. had seen in many a year. Still, I was very concerned. Somewhere, somehow, in the deep recesses of my mind, I *knew* I was dying.

Karen and I made daily calls to the Air Quality Management District (AQMD). One day, I reached a compassionate soul who told me about a biochemist named Dr. Erlander, who helped many people with this problem. At last, I thought, a human being who can help me! I phoned him. Obviously, a very bright man, he quickly filled me in on hydrocarbon allergy. ''With each time I ate an allergic food, thicker and thicker mucous was forming in my intestines. Day by day, I would ''lose'' more and more foods. ''The chemical load,'' he went on, ''from inhalant hydrocarbons, such as smog, would further contribute to my breakdown''. Eventually, I would fill with mucous and die. In shocked disbelief, I asked him what I could do. Briefly, he outlined his program which eliminated hydrocarbons and introduced a planned allergy diet which tricks the immune system, allowing it to heal and function properly. I thought he was nuts, thanked him for his advice, and hung up ·badly shaken.

There must be some easy answer, I told myself. I returned to Lisot and asked for lung studies to check my status there. Breathing tests show obstruction or lung disease. A Dr. Gibb, a colleague of Dr. Lisot, did respiratory tests, without drugs, via my request. Puzzled, he said ''The tests show a hypersensitivity of the vagus nerve, a major nerve to all the internal organs . . '' But he didn't know what it meant or how to help me. A native of Berkeley, he advised me against the move, as that area was the allergy capital of the world. Of course, I thanked him for his concern, and ignored what he said.

My private life continued to be a mess. Wanting to get on with life, I signed up for an 18-month certification course as a financial planner. This would keep my mind off all my problems, I mused, and be a giant step toward insuring my future. In the meantime, the anaphylactic reactions increased. Trying to get rid of cellulite on the back of my upper legs, I used a body wrap in a friend's figure salon. Anaphylaxis resulted. Half-conscious, I barely made it in my car to Lisot's office, driving perilously. He looked scared and yelled at me, ''Elizabeth, be careful — this was almost it.'' ''It'' translated to death.

As a result of these experiences, I decided getting out of L.A. and away from Jean-Pierre would solve my problems. I flew to Berkeley and looked for a house to rent. Believed it was the right place to live.

Back to L.A. Nothing seemed to help me. Becoming more frightened every day, I was still afraid to move because my back dislocated very often and left me helpless. The thought of this occurring in a new city left me numb with fear. Yet I trekked on.

I told Jean-Pierre of my plans. He was very sad but agreed, for now I was beginning to lose consciousness when I drove the freeways. Although I finished my first class in financial planning, I handed in my resignation; the classroom was a basement room in a bank without air conditioning. I'd collapsed on the conference table twice. This was not meant for me.

By phone, I rented a professor's cottage in Berkeley for our six-weeks vacation in order to look for a permanent place. Delighted and optimistic about my solution, the girls and I prepared to debark to Berkeley for the months of July and August. The night before we left, I collapsed in the shower while shampooing my hair. We left anyway.

I never felt right from the moment I arrived. Yet, it was better than L.A. Forest fires had the Berkeley air polluted with smoke. I figured the smoke was the problem and would pass.

One evening, I joined several people in a restaurant. It was filled with cigarette smoke. Chest pain began quietly, in my right lung. *Oh no, not again — not like Maui.* It had been almost five years since this had happened.

Stoically, I drove home. The pain was so severe I could hardly breathe. I phoned a new acquaintance, a fine woman, Nina, and begged her for help. She rushed over. My color must have been awful for she called an ambulance. This even frightened brave me. In the emergency room, they wanted to do arterial blood gases. Novacaine is necessary, for the test is severely painful. I told them I was allergic to Novacaine (had shock last time I'd been administered this anesthetic). The alert physician said, ''I'll use sterile sodium chloride — has the same effect.'' He felt it was an embolus. *God no — not that diagnosis again.* The Emergency physician called in a cardiovascular specialist. Dr. Zeb listened to my story till 5:00A.M. He didn't know what to make of me, for the blood gas was negative and that usually clinches the diagnosis. At one point, they gave me a minute dose of Demerol subcutaneously, as I'd instructed them I was recovering from chemical addiction. A crying jag ensued. I didn't connect the two.

I was admitted to a regular room. Within hours, my body had a red rash all over it. Sheets? Drugs? No one knew. The nurse called the doctor. He ordered benadryl, an antihistamine for allergic reactions.

The next day I phoned Jean-Pierre and made arrangements to fly the girls back to Santa Monica where he would take care of them during my hospitalization. I really loved him for this. The doctor released me three days later. I spent the last two weeks of my vacation alone, barely able to move, for the exhaustion was extreme now. Somehow, in my few good moments, I was able to rent a lovely house in the Berkeley Hills.

I flew back to Santa Monica and prepared to leave for a week on Vancouver Island, Canada with Jean-Pierre. Elatedly I said, ''We can celebrate your divorce which will be tomorrow.'' Sheepishly, he looked at me — ''I'm sorry but I have bad news for you. I have to stay married this year for tax reasons.'' My heart sunk; my gut raged. After screaming at him I decided to go on the trip anyway and enjoy the scenic town. At this point I decided to let Jean-Pierre go completely when we returned, as the relationship had nowhere to go, and I was being hurt more and more every day. It's obvious by now, I'm a highly capable person able to handle many things at once. That would all change.

The week in Victoria was glorious. Well, all the time, with the exception of an anaphylactic reaction in a smoke filled restaurant. The memory of this wonderful week was going to have to sustain me for a long time to come.

Upon our return, I told Jean-Pierre it was all over between us; the deceit and stalling had changed my feelings for him. I realized he had a long way to go before he was free emotionally and physically of his failed marriage. With this, I bade him adieu. But he still hung around to help me a bit to prepare to leave.

Off to Berkeley on September 1st. Seems I wanted to leave behind many things. Jean-Pierre and I broke up. On my way to freedom and health — or so I erroneously thought.

My birthday would be September 18. A joyous occasion, full of the freedom of being one's own person; loneliness swept over me on my fifth day there. Neither mood mattered, for the terminal phase of the disease was upon me.

I believed I'd prepared myself well for my move — coming ahead a month early and establishing new friends and acquaintances both in and out of AA. Wrong, very wrong!

On September 8, I ate apple pan dowdy. Sugar I'd given up two years earlier. But the temptation proved too much. Four hours later, a suffocating feeling began and I became gray. I collapsed in front of my filter gasping for air. Terrified, I phoned Lisot. He referred me to a colleague in El Cerrito. ''Don't see your type of case,'' Dr. Burns said. ''Call Dr. Laura Best in Berkeley.'' Best was a clinical ecologist, a new term to me. She listened to my story, then said, ''You are too sick for me. I wouldn't be able to care for you, for I have the same disease but not in the severity you do. You are very ill. But I'll refer you to a doctor in Richmond.''

The next day, I saw Dr. Hall's partner, Dr. Arams. He heard my history, then said, ''We have hundreds of cases like yours. We can help you.'' Dr.

Arams gave me 12 pages of questions to answer at home and advised using a hypoallergenic shampoo. A battery of immune and allergy tests were also run. Oxygen was ordered for the mental confusion.

I returned on October 5th to Dr. Hall's office. His diagnosis was "Environmental illness with organic brain syndrome." What a diagnosis! By this he meant I had become "allergic" to the 20th Century — specifically all toxic substances — shampoo, soap, polyester, mattresses, gas heating, gas cooking, pine sol, car fumes, paint, tar, air pollution, etc. The list was over 2,000 substances that I was to avoid to stay alive. In essence, throw out your house, car, children and self, and you will be all right.

There had to be a mistake. In total emotional shock, I listened while in an anaphylactic reaction from the shampoo Dr. Arams had advised. The timing was poor. The cerebral anoxia (lack of oxygen) was so severe, I could hear him but not understand the words or respond. Brain toxicity causes these symptoms. *This one I could not survive alone.*

With this terrifyingly new development, I turned back to Jean-Pierre once more. He was very upset. "Come down, come down to L.A. so I can hold you." Confusion, love and hate streamed through me simultaneously. Not that dance of death again. But I needed him, so I acquiesced. Jean-Pierre's return to my life would prove crucial both in saving my sanity and in losing it. This indeed was Providence.

In 1981, the method for dealing with Environmental Illness was to do a battery of provocative allergy tests. "Clean" extracts were used (substances free of phenol, a member of the formaldehyde family which was a culprit in anaphylaxis). The tests were fine for persons in earlier stages of the disease.

Yet intuitively I knew this testing would kill me, for my body was past Western medicine's knowledge. Frightened beyond comprehension, I stumbled dazedly from Hall's office and drove home, realizing I was going to die. At this point I became hysterical, crying like a cornered animal. *What had I done to deserve this?* I raved at God, if there was one.

In my despair, I walked to the end of the Berkeley pier. I raged at God, "How could You do this to me?" I threatened suicide. Then I bargained with Him. "God, if you're out there, take away either this back problem or this illness." A peace descended upon me. From that day forth to this writing, my spine no longer dislocated; the problem was resolved. Awesome.

Returning home, I tried to get a grip on myself. Orthodox medicine had helped make me this sick; therefore, I reasoned, unorthodox medicine had to provide new answers.

Somewhere in this blurring whirl of horror, someone presented me with the information that there was a support group in San Francisco for this problem. Grateful, I phoned several numbers.

They were very hopeless about my condition. Finally, I reached a woman named Eve Bergman, a compassionate soul who would become very instrumental in saving my life for she had been there.

Terrified of Dr. Hall's approach, I re-phoned Dr. Best. She recommended Dr. Ray Cort, a physician in San Francisco. Immediately I phoned him. His assistant told me he had no openings for three weeks. I begged her to speak to him for an earlier appointment as I was deteriorating rapidly and felt I wouldn't live. She was very understanding and told me to keep in touch if I had any questions, that she'd call if there were any cancellations.

Lonely and afraid, I flew back to Los Angeles to spend a weekend with Jean-Pierre. He saw my fear and was very comforting. I was totally confused. *What brought this on? What could I do to help myself?* Not knowing the answers was driving me crazy. But I was determined to find them.

By the time I reached Cort on October 11, much had worsened. When I turned on the central gas heating in my house I felt faint and turned yellow. Each day I was unable to "tolerate" more and more foods. I also gave up smoking completely as the brain confusion and vertigo deepened.

It was probably the abrupt withdrawal from this potent hydrocarbon that completed the breakdown of my system (later on I discovered cigarettes have *111* chemicals *besides nicotine*), along with the spraying of malathion south of me around Palo Alto, which was carried by the winds to Berkeley. When I entered the street my head spun, my arms went numb, breathing became difficult and my body turned ashen; I had moved from a bad environment to a lethal one.

Desperately ill and terrified, I had a driver take me to Dr. Cort's office. We had an instant cameraderie. Again, I filled out eight pages of reactions to chemicals:

Caffeine — collapse.

Anesthesia — psychosis.

Diesel fumes — nausea and vomiting.

Perfume — headaches, hives, vomiting.

"You are one of the 30% with E.I. who have Candida. What Candida does," Cort went on, "is, untreated it eventually invades the bloodstream, sending at least 70 toxins to the hypothalamus in the brain, thereby causing mental aberrations such as anxiety, fear, paranoia, plus abnormal food and sex cravings (either hyper or hypo). The hypothalamus is the brain center controlling these functions. We have an experimental drug in yellow powder form, called nystatin, which we administer orally in ½ teaspoons, four times a day. When you take this drug, we hope the immune system will snap back after killing off the Candida, thereby enabling the immune system to come back and kill the fungus itself. In three months you will be well."

Though I didn't believe him, Cort gave me hope for the first time. An answer had been provided. Yet as a nurse, I'd worked with nystatin to rinse the Candida from the mouths of terminally ill cancer patients and had been warned thoroughly not to allow the patient to swallow it as it was a powerful drug.

I queried Cort on this fact. He said the present research showed this was the only available anti-fungal drug that was virtually non-toxic. Thinking back over my medical experience, I remembered reactions to other allegedly non-toxic drugs. This gave me pause. Cort said nystatin was my salvation; he also dubbed me a "universal reactor". "I'll go home and think it over."

Go home, I did. Immediately, I phoned Eve. "Yes, I've been on it about a year and I've improved greatly. But it does have side effects, Elizabeth — bloating, weight gain and joint pain." *She was still alive, so she must have done something right.*

Eve also told me Dr. Orion Truss in Birmingham, Alabama was the undisclosed world expert on Candida. "Perhaps you could give him a call." Eve's loving voice did more for my state of mind than any drug could have.

I weighed both opinions. Still, an inner voice told me in my present state of toxicity nystatin would cause my demise. Taking it didn't feel right, so I decided to detox gradually as I'd been instructed by Eve.

Meanwhile, the lengthy symptomatology list Dr. Cort had me fill out brought back memories. The psychoses, after the birth of both children — From nowhere appeared fear and paranoia. In one instance, blades of grass on a cliffside became flames coming to get me. The night sweats. The thyroid pills. That was it! With my first child, the obstetrician had given me thyroid for the fatigue during the pregnancy. When I figured it out myself, and stopped the thyroid, the symptoms immediately disappeared. The second pregnancy, after toxic doses of carbocaine (doctor informed me), a suicidal depression developed. Thinking it was caused solely by my child's birth defects, I signed myself into a private psychiatric hospital. Diagnosed as "psychotic" by the psychiatrist, he placed me on Thorazine. Knowing drugs' side-effects extremely well, I demanded I be taken off this drug. Purple crusts had formed on my eyelids while I was also crawling along the hospital walls trying to stand up. Being on the other side of insanity, not the nurse in charge, was a whole experience in itself. The dehumanization of a human to a label — "psychotic" — was placed on me. I hated it. Two weeks was all I could stand. I signed myself out. Perhaps, I had a nervous break-down. I suspect it was chemically induced.

The severe nausea and vomiting through both pregnancies floated before my eyes and the cravings . . . . The cravings for carbohydrates were maddening . . . . And the vomiting . . . . Passing out from one sip of alcohol . . . . It all made sense now . . . . The mosaic was coming together . . . .

ISOLATION

In October of '81, I began changing my diet to organic, non-pesticide sprayed foods. Now the horror really began. Anaphylaxis from everything — the bed, the clothes, the food, the air and the bottled water. Over the next three weeks, anaphylactic reactions claimed my soul almost day and night. They have a definite pattern: severe mental confusion, feeling one is dying (not fainting) as the energy drains right from the top of your head out your toes, severe shaking chills, exhaustion, physical collapse, semi-consciousness, in and out of a gray fog, slurred speech, leaden body, inability to move, and finally total helplessness. This is followed by cerebral toxicity — fear, paranoia, and horrifying hallucinations (voices) which can conclude in death. Fortunately (?), my reaction only went to the very edge of annihilation and stayed there. Despair and weeping uncontrollably comes as the reaction ends. It lasts five minutes, five hours or five days. The terror is unspeakable.

My health, my life were going. Just changing the diet was killing me. So I stopped. Once again, I trusted my inner voice. *Slowly Elizabeth, very slowly, make these changes in your life.* The healing of this illness is long term. Strongly, I believed I would be healed completely. All I had to learn was how.

Once more in desperation, I turned to Eve. She verified my thoughts. "Progress very slowly Elizabeth, change one thing at a time and give yourself two to four weeks for your body to adjust." Excellent advice. Eve was so anxious to help that she bombarded me with suggestions on herbs and vitamins. On her suggestion I tried kelp. Turned yellow and collapsed in shock. Taken to emergency room by an acquaintance. Doctors didn't know how to treat me . . . . used only oxygen . . . . recovered three hours later spontaneously. . . .

Obviously, what worked for Eve did not work for me. When I recovered fully, I phoned to tell her what had happened. ''Oh my,'' she replied, ''You'd better not do anything for awhile, just adjust to the diet.''

During October, more horrifying symptoms were added to my body. One morning as I was putting on mascara, gray mucous poured from my eyes, blurring my vision. Totally lost the ability to wash my hair with any shampoo, lemon, or eggs. Shock. A special filter placed over the shower head removing chlorine, permitted me to ''rinse'' my body. Chest and arm pain when I touched the telephone; ''lost'' voice too. Shock, if my children entered my bedroom with perfume scent on their hair picked up from school; shock, when my nurse's aide cooked on the new electric stove the floor below. Normal scents became one-hundred times normal, smelling only petrochemical odor in the substance. Entire body bright red if I tried to wear nylon or turned on the new electric heater. Shock. One side of my body was blue tinged, the other waxen when I attempted to attend the Environmental Illness monthly meeting at a local church. Shock, always shock, now, accompanied every reaction. Couldn't ''tolerate'' life.

I cannot describe the demoralization of a human being who cannot bathe, use deodorant, or wash her hair.

The weight loss continued till my clothes hung off me. I lived in an old pair of cotton jeans and blouse for nine months — these were the only clothes I didn't go into shock from. I was physically unable to buy any. My face was waxen and covered with red blotches. My hair hung in stringy, greasy strands. Despair became my continual look. The only soap I could tolerate on planet earth was handmade of pure olive oil by Dr. Erlander, the biochemist. Every time I phoned him in my hopeless state, he reiterated — ''Get rid of the bed. The bedding companies'' he related, ''use multiple toxic chemicals to preserve the mattress and retard burning. My research shows these chemicals still haven't gassed out after thirty years.'' I thought he was nuts. I didn't listen.

Christmas was drawing near. New toxins further imprisoned me. People in the Berkeley Hills are fond of their fireplaces. So fond, in fact they burn many poisonous substances, such as plastics, in the fire besides wood. Woodsmoke for this environmentally ill person was lethal. The first smell turned my body yellow. Severe chest pain (pulmonary vasculitis) followed the inhalation along with brain insanity from the toxic fumes. Slam. Locked the windows to keep out the deadly fumes; locked myself in for the winter period. I'd be a liar if I didn't say I contemplated suicide over and over. All I had to do was dye my hair and it would be all over.

Hydrocarbon poisoning in this form is endless. After sealing all the windows in my bedroom with aluminum foil, and stripping it to the bare necessities — a bed, lamp and nightstand — a new threat reared its ugly head. Mold, at this stage of candidiasis, triggers suicidal depressions that are so exaggerated as to be compared to a person who has drunk a fifth of vodka and is in a suicidal crying jag. Blackouts began while driving. Mold. Had to hire a full time driver.

Doomed. Suicidal depressions, shock, life-threatening vasculitis in the form of excruciating chest pain. Couldn't read, write, watch T.V., or listen to the radio. In this terminal stage, the body cannot tolerate the slightest toxic fumes — everything becomes life-threatening. To say I was living a living death, is an understatement.

The dying comes slowly at this point. Ten pounds underweight, living on distilled water and six vegetables plus organic turkey was how far down I'd gone in three months. Besides all this, I was surviving a freezing winter without heat of any kind because I went into shock from every kind of heater. I decided to tell my children I was dying and ask them if they wanted to go live with their father. "No," both said. "We'll stay with you, Mom." My family on the East Coast had their own problems and could not take them. Divorce had stripped me of most of my old life and, with it, the old acquaintances and friends. They were too far away. My ex-husband said if he took them, he'd not return them. I could sink no lower. I slammed the phone in his ear. Life seemed hopeless.

The breakdown was so severe by Christmas of '81 I could barely leave my home. Still, with Jean-Pierre's assistance I was able to fly to L.A. for the holidays. A precarious, terrifying trip at best, now knowing planes are full of formaldehyde, pesticides, diesel fumes, and cigarette smoke. L.A.'s air was better, believe it or not, than Berkeley's because it was drier and relatively free of mold. I had a home in Santa Monica which I'd rented out for a year while I lived in Berkeley. So I stayed at Jean-Pierre's. No other human being can understand this disease, for one has to live it to believe it. Jean-Pierre did the best he could but couldn't handle the anger and rage out of nowhere. Our relationship resembled a razor's edge.

Right before my return to Berkeley on New Year's Day, in a "mold," suicidal depression, I wrote a despairing letter to God:

Dear God,

I'm writing you again because Your child's spirit is so broken. I know I must be humbled but this is a little heavy handed.

I'm having trouble making it through today. Friends visited and I loved it, but perfume fumes almost annihilated me.

I don't know where to go
I don't know what to do
I don't have any answers
And I am in despair

I can't live in Berkeley. I can't live here. It's all very simple. I tried going it locked up and I wasn't making it.

My reserve seems gone
Where is the strength you promised me?

Where is the help? It takes all I've got to survive
I'm a fighter but this one is destroying me
Tonight I'm going under again.
Trying to relieve the chest pain.
Filter on, air machine, window open
For once, people can't help
Please give me some help
    Its all I ask
    For my despair is total
I can not face returning to Berkeley alone and sick
I cannot lose my money to live on
I cannot take care of my children
Life is a burden
I'm too sick and overwhelmed
Where is the legs I was promised?
What am I going to do? My time here is
limited and nowhere to go

I have money, means and nowhere to go
Should I try nystatin?
Whom should I trust?
Is Erlander the answer?

I'm afraid to go on like this
Life is very isolated, very sick
Where are You?
Where is a safe place?

How could You have done this to me?

Jean-Pierre comes home from work exhausted to this?
It's not that I feel a burden to people, I just can't go on
    The reaction's all day like an ongoing nightmare

If I knew I was dying, it would be easier — I'd enjoy life until I
dropped, but what can you do to enjoy life if you are constantly
reminded by normal people you are isolated, different, bizarre?

I write all my despair to You because it's the way I feel tonight

And so God, if it's not in Your plan to give me a break, then take
me 'cause I can't live with the daily collapsing, half blacking out,
chest pain, feeling like I'm dying, inability to be near other people.
    I'm begging you like an animal about to be quartered
    I cannot take any more
    Thank you for all the love and people You sent me — I'll
remember them
    I've been through a lot and I don't understand why or how

All I have to do is wash my hair or turn on the stove
or eat ice cream
Crazy way to go but then I can't believe You'd make anyone this
sick and expect them to go on living — it doesn't make sense
All my friends are here and I feel good about that
Although my strength comes and goes

Will You ask me what step was I working when I committed
suicide?
Where is my faith? Have I not suffered enough, the tortures of
the damned, have I not been through enough?
I am mortal and very aware of it at this moment.
So where are You?
I've given myself to You
I cannot change my fate. I've done my best.

Take me

Elizabeth Rose
December 28, 1981
10:30pm

The sun shone brightly the next morning. Jean-Pierre flew with me
back to Berkeley. The mold was gone. That evening, I turned on the electric
heater. *Nothing happened.* Coincidence, or had God heard my prayers?
''Nothing happened'' would become a familiar phrase in my recovery.

To make it simpler for you, I've decided to divide recovery into three chapters: physical, mental, and spiritual. The combinations healed me, especially the latter. Until this time, this part of my existence was denied. It would prove to be the most crucial in my recovery.

PART II

THE RECOVERY

PHYSICAL

There is a natural progression in the healing of candidiasis at the final stage that is essential: Learning early on that the physical healing must be slow and consistent with one's state of mind. By this I mean that while one is changing one's entire diet, one must also continuously tell oneself, "I will be well," in between cerebral reactions. Survival is what we want, then a return to living. This takes time and a great deal of patience.

I found changing the diet had to be done over a six-month period. From October till May I moved very slowly. This gives the body time to adjust to a radical change of diet gently. Most Candida sufferers at this stage have no diet per se — many are living on nuts and ice cream — the two foods E.I.'s crave, which feed Candida. Alcohol is also craved by those with this predeliction or a family history of alcoholism.

First of all, I encourage you to go to a qualified physician and be diagnosed. A special immune panel will help uncover this hidden ailment. The tests are: Ig series (immune system), T and B lymphocytes count, prostaglandins, and liver chemistries.

Secondly, special filters free of ozone clean up indoor pollution. I was able to tolerate the Faust all-metal model. It probably saved my life many times when my body was blasted by a chemical. I'd kneel on the floor and stick my nose in it, sucking up the clean air. This filter was also excellent at unpolluting the atmosphere in a matter of minutes. A filter combined with air conditioning (portable units, not central, which are full of chemicals and gas residual) produces a relatively fresh-aired oasis.

An oasis is very important. I set up one room in my house — my bedroom with wooden floors — which I stripped of everything. Borax was placed in cups in the closets to keep the mold under control. The oasis can be the life-saving factor in a crisis. *I cannot recommend this strongly enough*.

Most clinical ecologists will recommend a rotation diet whereby you make a five-day menu plan, not using the same food twice for four to five days. Allegedly, this reduces allergic responses. Not believing this illness to be ''allergy'' per se, but a toxic breakdown of the immune system, I skeptically tried it from October '81 till March of '82. I quickly learned I was allergic to almost every food and did not have enough foods to rotate. Now what does one do? I also lived on distilled water. Spring water's high natural salt content induced shock in me. The rotation diet is overwhelming when one is this ill for I was unable to cook or stand up at this point, and hired help to live in for a small sum.

Just to survive, I had the same food cooked in large batches early in the morning, then picked at it all day. On the rotation diet, I became more and more sensitive to grains and fruits with little or no improvement in my status. All fruit juices made me dizzy and faint.

What was going on here? I asked myself. From the rotating diet, I was deteriorating. Time for Eve. She suggested bicarbonate of soda or Alka-Seltzer Gold to stop the food reactions. I tried some and became very ill — collapse, mental confusion, entire insides felt on fire. The diet produced a new symptom — asthma. What next?

The asthma resulted from sesame butter which was recommended to me in place of regular butter. Peanuts was the food I craved continuously. I would eat three eight-ounce bags in one sitting and produce peanut butter as an end product. And keep losing weight! Sugar, I thought I'd given up two years earlier but found it hidden in many foods — especially those commercially prepared.

Rapidly I discovered, any food with chemical preservatives or sprayed with pesticides could not be ''tolerated'' at all. In our present day toxic world, that left almost nothing.

Dr. Hall also recommended I go to the beach daily, or to move there for clean air. Since I couldn't stand up or drive, this was a ludicrous suggestion. And I soon discovered crossing the Oakland Bay Bridge could be lethal when caught in a traffic jam. (Air currents around bridges lock in the fuel emissions, thereby increasing one's reactions.) Upon entering the bridge, with a friend driving, my color was gray. I also learned from the San Francisco AQMD that fog and cold winter air hold hydrocarbons to the ground. At rush hour, from 3:30 'til 7pm, the amount of hydrocarbons in the air is increased tenfold. No wonder I collapsed in this ''clean air.'' Positive ions (hydrocarbon) are the destroyers of the immune system. By depressing it, the body becomes more vulnerable to illness. Negative ions are the body's healers. The doctors believed they were at the ocean.

Finally, I hired a lovely woman to drive me to the beach. We arrived. I immediately turned yellow, saw black spots, had severe nausea, and felt my head was being crushed in a vise. Obviously the ocean, at this point in time, would not aid my recovery.

A ray of hope finally came in December of '81. While visiting Santa Monica, I decided to re-consider Dr. Erlander as a possible solution to this nightmare. An appointment made, Jean-Pierre drove me to Pasadena to Stig's little cubbyhole. He interviewed me in the street with portable oxygen running, for I could not physically "tolerate" his office quarters.

"Yes, I can help you." He explained thoroughly about hydrocarbon allergy. For a fee, he gave me a taped program, booklet, and all his assistance by phone.

At the same time, while still in L.A., Jean-Pierre and I took advantage of the clean cool winter air and decided to find a place for me to live with unpolluted air. Erlander suggested Pearblossom between L.A. and Vegas. We placed this on our itinerary. Oxygen, car filter, and carbon mask in tow, we began our trek looking for an environment in which I could heal.

We tried Pearblossom first. The name itself was hilarious; the town was even more so. Stuck out somewhere on Interstate 405. We came to a gas station and a grocery store. That was it — with the exception of about ten run-down houses. There was nothing in either direction for miles. Yes, the air was clean. But the place was isolated. And I'd be alone. Terror. Jean-Pierre was not willing to come with me. His career was more important.

Pearblossom provided great material for a taping on our return trip. I "interviewed" Jean-Pierre about Pearblossom, asking his opinion. He burped into the microphone. "That sums it up folks." All Jean-Pierre could do was laugh about Pearblossom. He was speechless. We snapped a picture so we'd never forget it. Even in the picture the town wasn't quite there. We were told the temperature went from 115° to 13° — below zero. We laughed ourselves back to L.A. The Polaroid mainly failed in Pearblossom because it was too cold to take a picture.

The next day, we drove down the Southern California coast. I taped the journey for the benefit of other E.I. sufferers. Here is my research:

1) Malibu — heavy mold and fog most of the year, Candida patients seem to be sickest here.
2) Santa Monica — pockets of clean air, best about 1 mile from beach.
3) Torrance and Redondo Beach — refineries, severe suicidal depressions — unliveable
3) Wilmington - Long Beach — refineries severe suicidal depressions — unliveable
5) Cardiff-by-the-Sea — clean air and low mold problem — good air currents — wood smoke in winter — some electric houses — didn't seem to get much fog. Santa Ana occasionally. (Had bagel and croissant store — almost sold me on this town.)
6) Leucadia — light smog — moldy — better up above the beach on the bluff.

7) Encinitas — severe mold reactions at beach — unliveable — more in a valley inland — clear, cooler and good — a lot of nurseries — heavy smell of bleach
8) Carlsbad — chemical smell — farmland nearby — not good
9) Tamarack — power plant giving off fumes
10) Oceanside — heavy car fumes (rush hour). Chemical smell here too. More inland — more densely populated.
11) San Onofre — power plant — air heavy, smelled of chemicals, trapped.

A big clue to the diagnosis is provided here if one becomes ill at the beach. I'd strongly suspect candidiasis. I'd also be careful about buying or renting a house in a shady area, for mold problems are greatly exaggerated in this atmosphere.

This survey was conducted at various hours of the day, so car fumes have to be taken into consideration. However, a large area of Southern California is covered with a great deal of farmland and one must stop to consider the effect of the pesticides being used on the air quality. Needless to say, Santa Monica seemed the only liveable place for me.

Back in Berkeley, I shortly realized the diet wasn't "tolerated" by my body. Erlander detoxes you by placing you on vegetables and potatoes for four days. The food cravings drove me to eat ten potatoes in one day. My abdomen swelled as if I were eight months pregnant. Exhaustion and collapse. Stig seemed puzzled. "No one has gotten that sick." Intuitively, again, I knew his program was not the complete answer.

But it was *part* of the solution. Gently but firmly, he told me each phone call, "Get rid of the bed you're sleeping on." I ignored him — he was exaggerating I told myself. Advising me to change all my utensils to stainless steel, and steaming my food in bottled water reduced hydrocarbon overload. And last but not least, Dr. Erlander taught me to cook green vegetables in a crock pot using bottled spring water. This procedure neutralized the acid and the water became alkaline, which enabled me to obtain minerals for my system through drinking the vegetable water. In this fashion, I could tolerate bottled spring water. As a direct result of his recommendations, I could eat more vegetables. I give him a lot of credit for saving my life.

Erlander also explained acid - alkaline base to me from a scientist's viewpoint. Acid people, such as myself, have the most severe reactions but the best capacity for rapid healing; alkaline people heal more slowly and have less severe chemical reactions.

He also taught me to test my saliva and urine with nitrazine paper which one can buy from him at a nominal price. You placed the paper under your tongue when in a reaction. If it reads acid, eat something alkaline; if the reverse, eat an acid food. Keeping the acid-alkaline base balanced is crucial to healing. The normal Ph of urine is 7, and blue on the nitrazine paper. Acid registers yellow. Registering yellow means you are in a continuous reaction and very ill. I was "yellow." Knowing these simple facts began the turn-around in my illness — the beginning of healing, for Stig had given me guidelines to work with.

Eventually, I listened to him about the toxic bed. Calling around to second hand stores in my collapsed state, I located an old dark green, folding iron bed. I made a mattress from woolen and cotton blankets. *Immediately felt better getting off my bed.* As soon as I lay on my bed again, my heart pounded, I became agitated, turned red, got shocky, depressed and weepy. *He was right.*

The winter mold made my bedroom unliveable. Now began living in my bathroom for the next six months — a strange, wild, funny, sad experience.

With the hydrocarbon load lessened in my cooking and bedding, my brain had some clarity. However, due to the heavy mold in Berkeley, my body could not tolerate Erlander's diet which he said requires a mold-free environment. But I survived this letdown and lived to laugh about it the next day.

February 23, 1982. The Berkeley air is clear. I'm not reacting on chemicals. So clean air does help! But where to live? The last move physically was the completion of my breakdown. No, moving was not the answer.

Daily walks told me my physical condition. If I could walk the Berkeley pier in 20 minutes, I was in good shape; in an hour or unable at all, a poor day. Exercise is imperative, even if it's for two minutes an hour. Toxins are released from the body this way. Since I'd stopped sweating almost a year ago, releasing toxins from my body was very difficult. Eve had mentioned a portable trampoline, which I've used only recently due to my poor condition and inability to tolerate physically the material it was made from. The trampoline stimulates the lymph glands which are the body's filtration system, thereby rinsing out the toxins.

Let me mention here how difficult I found it to stick with any one regime. The more one investigates, the more one runs into conflicting theories. Before Erlander, I'd tried hypnosis to reduce the chemical reactions. In discussing this with Stig, he felt it was dangerous because it could knock out the second immune system (humoral) by reducing the histamine level of the body. I tended to agree with him and gave that up. My critical condition eliminated moving again; it prompted me to look for another answer. Eve gently recommended trying nystatin once again. By this time terror was my everyday companion and I feared anything new being placed in my body. So I called Steve Levine, a biochemist and fellow E.I. sufferer, for his advice. Nystatin had helped his healing. After listening to my story he said, "Elizabeth you're one of the mold people. Nystatin will heal you. You don't have to move or do anything. You're a prime candidate for the drug and will be well and able to live anywhere." My hopes soared as a result of this conversation. I'm deeply grateful to him to this very day for his uplifting advice.

Between January and March, I lived on a roller coaster. My illness was a never-ending clarity — insanity trip, not knowing when the madness or the physical symptoms would strike, no matter what I did. I also broke up with and reconciled with Jean-Pierre every other week. My life was sheer madness. The time was coming for me to consider nystatin, for I couldn't go on this way.

Deciding to take nystatin wasn't easy. I knew it had some serious side effects from talking to fellow E.I.s, but what were my choices? A momentous event in my life on March 2, cemented in my brain the courage to try this experimental drug. The event was recorded by me as a "Vignette from the Berkeley Pier".

"Elizabeth stood despairingly at the walkway to the pier. The sun slept peacefully while the cold March wind pierced each molecule of her body. *Stop voices, stop, stop telling me to jump off.* The illness is winning, screeching, *end it, end it.* Her brain bursting with chemical reactions from the moldy air, *can't bear another moment.* Her soul screams out to God, "Help me, help me, I don't want to die." Her emotions exploding in her mind say *fishermen of the pier, help me. I'm insane from this illness and I can't stop the voices in my head, seducing me to certain death.*

But she speaks not a word. Her despair is total. For six months Elizabeth has lived in a two-story house with her two daughters, Amy and Jen, surviving the ravages of a nightmarish disease presently named "E.I." This monstrous phenomenon is a product of 20th century man's "progress" — the introduction of plastics and pesticides and chemicals into the environment which insidiously cause a collapse of the immune system and the host becomes toxic to everything in life — clothes, food, perfumes, synthetics, fabrics, gas fumes, paint and cleansers, to name a few. In order to survive, doctors order all of these be removed from the environment to allow the body to repair.

Unfortunately, life is not as perfect as the doctors wish, and this severe isolation from human touch and caring, plus the mad brain reactions, had led Elizabeth to the pier for her demise.

Quietly, she strolls the mile-long pier wanting to cry out for help, too far gone to ask. Straight ahead she sees a very tall, slim man, around 30 walking before her with his catch for the day. *Any human contact will do Elizabeth, any.* Anxiously she hastens her pace, hoping he will notice her, until, she passes him on the pier. Almost like a movie plot, he approaches her and speaks "Come here very often?"

"Everyday when the air is clear" Elizabeth replies, as her mind continues fragmenting.

"When the air is clear?" he queries perplexed.

"Yes," holding back the tears, "I'm seriously ill and clean air is my only hope of healing."

The tide of tears follows. She cannot speak. Tears roll from under her deep purple sunglasses.

"Hey," he says, "is it that bad?"

"Yes," she tells the handsome 6'4" stranger.

"I came here to jump off."

"Are you serious?" he replied compassionately

"I am." And the tears pour as from a deep well, newly discovered.

"Come here," he said gently, "and sit on these rocks with me, and we can talk."

"But you're a stranger," she said fearfully.

"Sometimes it's the best way."

"Do you have any scent on?"

"No, just came back from my house in Clearwater Lake — just me — that's all."

Feeling a bit more comfortable, Elizabeth sits on a gray rock across from him, crying and saying to herself — *What am I doing with a stranger — telling him my despair. Am I so desperate for human kindness I will take it from a stranger? Yes I will. He was sent to me for a reason.*

He wanted to know more. She spilled the horror story out and left it lying in his lap like a tub of pus.

But he didn't run, or become frightened as the others had. No.

He said, "I've been through a similar event in my life. I was shot down in Viet Nam and spent six weeks in a coma. Apparently, I was told, I put a nurse's eye out in a violent seizure, of which I have no recollection. I still feel badly about that. I wish I could find her and do something to help her." Then he related how he returned to the states and couldn't finish college because his brain retention of new material had been damaged. He also had no recollection of his life before the accident. So he said, he'd learned to go slowly, dabble at photography, and enjoy fishing and friends.

So he had suffered too.

"My only hope is taking nystatin," I told him, "An antifungal drug that can kill me while it kills the candida."

"Take it," he said. "What have you got to lose? I'm sure you'll be all right." That statement made up my mind for me. This stranger was giving me hope.

Elizabeth was curious now.

"How old are you?"

"Thirty," he said. "And you?"

Cagily, Elizabeth replied, "older than you."

"You look about 25 with hair prematurely graying."

Elizabeth, who'd been a beauty, whose vanity had been totally humbled by this experience, who could no longer touch up the gray, confessed she was 30ish. He was amazed and reached out to touch her uncosmetiqued face, saying, "You are a natural beauty"

Elizabeth was feeling alarm at this turn of events while enjoying being flirted with. Almost no attention for six months and having to relinquish her glamour girl status left her vaguely vulnerable and uneasy with herself.

As her discomfort grew, Elizabeth abruptly bolted from the rock, brusquely turned around and stared straight into the sun glowing on the murky water.

Let him look and enjoy a great beauty she said to herself smugly.

"You're built like a brick s... house, woman." This further titillated and annoyed her.

"I'm going to walk the pier again. My legs are numb from sitting," she said paranoid, wanting to end the encounter. Isolated from people for six months, she now realized had had a devastating effect on her psyche.

"Mind if I come along." Yes and no, she said concurrently to herself and him. Her vulnerability was exposed to both of them.

"I'd like to take you to my cabin in Clearwater. I'll take care of you." He meant it.

How presumptuous she retorted, to herself *doesn't he realize we are worlds apart?* Then her fear softened, knowing she was just like him, in need of a friend, and the hiatus no longer existed.

"I'd like to photograph you," he said, drinking in her large almond-shaped, gray-green eyes with endless lights dancing deliciously. The paleness of her face only accented her vulnerability. Yet she felt on very weak ground: a part wanted to be held and loved, another saying, careful, this pain shall pass. The man continued in his blatant seduction but she no longer heard him. She felt much relieved making contact with another human being, and knew that was all she needed.

Elizabeth became impatient to disengage from him. Grateful, so grateful for his kindness but she was too afraid to tell him. He wanted to see her again.

Perhaps — at the pier. "My name is James." "O.K. James."

He offered her his perch. Graciously, she declined.

Her spirit was sated. Alive again, she once more felt strengthened to fight, to survive.

She watched him leave and walk to his orange Toyota. Then with a final glance at the water, knowing the gift she'd been given, Elizabeth thanked God and went home.

The next day I began nystatin.

NYSTATIN THERAPY

On March 3, 1982, I stepped into Dr. Cort's office, terrified of taking nystatin, ready to take the step. For five days I'd attempted to hire a registered nurse to stay with me during the beginning phases of nystatin for I'd heard many horror stories about it and was unable to survive in a hospital.

Ray was funny. ''You won't die; I know emergency medicine. We'll give you adrenalin if necessary.''

''Adrenalin — it has phenol,'' I yelled at him hysterically, ''I'll croak.''

''Calm down, calm down.'' After listening carefully to Eve's advice about starting with a very small dose (gr 1/32), I told Cort, ''Skin test me for the drug.''

He mixed a sterile solution of approximately 1/1000 and injected it under my skin. Burning — but no other reaction. Good. Encouraged, I drank approximately 1/64 of a teaspoon of the bright yellow liquid. Severe dizziness descended upon me. I felt faint. Panic set in. ''Relax, relax, I'm here,'' he reassured me. I really needed to hear that. The symptoms resolved. My aide-driver took me home.

One hour later everything started to go black in front of my eyes. I almost passed out. Stumbling, I fell on my bed feeling high, giddy, and drunk plus exhaustion. My eyes and nose running. A feeling of lead as if I were anesthetized, permeated my body. Cort called at exactly this time.

''How are you?''

''Drunk,'' I replied giddily in slurred speech.

''Great, great,'' he blurted out joyously. ''It's working — you're on your way. Expect to feel the worst on the fourth day. Call me if you have any problems.''

Never in my life had I felt so grateful for a physician as I did at that moment.

My symptoms were relieved from the first dose! Dizziness, nausea and headaches (similar to motion sickness) appeared 2½ hours after the first dose. I had taken gr 1/32 — a minimal dose. By 5pm, I was coherent and felt wonderful and so it continued.

The next two days were the same — collapsing from 2-5pm, then okay. The fourth day was as predicted. In my journal, I recorded these notes:

> ''I felt dizzy and weak after my morning dose then increasingly weak and 'stoned' (drunk), became leaden by 2pm, recovered at 5pm and went under again from 6-7:30pm.''

It was hard to believe. *This was it!* I felt wonderful. A list of symptoms were relieved in just days:

1) Severe depression and suicidal thinking.
2) Mental confusion, disorientation as to place and why I'm there.
3) Water intolerance (bottled).
4) Hands reddening and pounding around television.
5) Chest pain and tightness around perfume and gas fumes.
6) Egg and butter allergy.
7) Chronic crying at 4 to 6pm daily.
8) Severe mental disturbances in rain and fog.
9) No collapsing, anger or rage from perfume.

This week, beginning nystatin, had turned my life around. Alleluia!

Jean-Pierre arrived at 4pm, smelling of scent and smoke, which he'd picked up in his hair from the airplane, to celebrate the good news. I gabbed with him through a carbon mask outside the house, until a shower was available (kids occupied both bathrooms). Usually, he had to climb through the ground floor bathroom window, strip his contaminated clothes, and shower in Aloe Vera shampoo and Erlander's olive soap before he could come near me.

Despite his decontamination in the shower, Jean-Pierre still had scent on his hair which we determined was residual hairspray. The help had to wash all his clothing in baking soda so he could wear them around me. We retired to my bedroom, the oasis. His eyes began running and *he* felt weak. I became weak and depressed. Mold. *That was the culprit.* Unfortunately, a side effect of nystatin is increased sensitivity to molds and mold foods. The bedroom was affecting me too! Upon leaving that room, both of our symptoms cleared up.

That day Berkeley was fogged in, rainy and moldy — my deadly enemies — plus wood smoke — *and I felt terrific.* Jean-Pierre cried when he first embraced me, seeing that my color had improved and I was beginning to look human again. So happy was he to see me healing that we commemorated the event by driving to a nearby Plaza and picking out a delayed Christmas present for Amy, a St. Patrick's Day prayer of luck for Jean-Pierre in his new job, and pink roses for me. A joyous half-hour. At home we danced to music. Jean-Pierre photographed me. Simple, warm, lovely. Impossible before nystatin.

That evening we cuddled in my green, iron, folding bed in the bathroom after multiple interruptions by the girls. Jean-Pierre began crying. We held each other tightly. He was so relieved I was going to be okay that he could finally allow himself to fall apart. Said he was lonely — worked, worked, worked to escape what was happening both in my life and his. He needed hugs for once which I gave him freely. This was followed by a fine meal of laughter, talking, love notes, chicken, spinach and rice.

Confidence entered my life again. Alive once more, I rushed out and ate foods I hadn't for a long time. Plus exposed myself to car fumes and some polyester. Food cravings descended upon me worse than ever. Nuts were the only food that sated my hunger. Tons of them. Eve to the rescue. ''The nystatin causes hypoglycemia with the candida die-off.'' Mine had been severe before treatment; it became the same in recovery, only in shorter intervals. ''A complete protein will alleviate the symptoms,'' Eve advised — ''I use alfalfa sprouts in mid-afternoon before the 4 o'clock slump.'' I tried it and it worked! All I had to do was adjust my diet a little bit.

On the seventh day of taking nystatin, I noticed more changes for the better: reading was slowly returning, could watch TV, windows open all night with wood smoke and nothing happened, and only reacted slightly to scent on my lawyer's witness when they visited that afternoon.

I conferred with Eve regularly now rather than my doctor, for he'd only told me to try the ''Cave Man'' diet which is vegetables, fruits, nuts and grains. Eve mentioned the candida diet which was just coming out of Dr. Truss's office in Alabama.

I couldn't believe this diet! Essentially, exist on vegetables (except starchy ones such as potatoes and sweet potatoes) fish, and chemically free meats and fowl. No fruit, dairy, grains or yeast, pickled or smoked foods. Already virtually reduced to non-eating, recovery from E.I. required even more rigid, limited eating. Yet, some foods had come back for me by now (all chemically free). But I did notice fruit was out for within 20 minutes after I ingested some, particularly apples, I had cerebrals, muscle tension in my jaw, throat and neck, and paranoia. Citrus guaranteed bleeding gums and herpes simplex within 24 hours. Were herpes and candida related? I began to think so. At this stage of recovery, I was still unable to tolerate vitamins or minerals but had gained the ability to drink bottled spring water. That was a vast improvement.

The tenth day on nystatin brought misery. My face turned red and burning. Numbness enveloped my hands, and cerebrals surfaced again — fear, paranoia, insanity, and depression. I felt as if I'd been through a war. Therefore, I increased the dosage a tiny bit. Everything started going black. Faint. Legs leaden. So I took another dose.

It felt like someone was ripping the inside of my head out through my teeth. Freaked, I called Cort, who told me to ''skip the next dose and take one at 10pm.'' The following day my body felt as if it had been run over by a truck. Exhaustion. Body ''bruised'' all over.

At the beginning of the second week of treatment I became bloated like a 5 months pregnant woman, and commenced passing large amounts of foul-smelling, green diarrhea stool and flatus. Now I was able to add cashew butter to my diet which was yummy and sated my food cravings — of course I ate the entire jar.

Two weeks into nystatin, I experienced mild flu symptoms. My dose remained at gr $\frac{1}{32}$ four doses daily. The only symptoms of the disease left were mild heachaches and nausea when exposed to fog, rain, woodsmoke, and tar all at once while walking in downtown Berkeley.

My adviser Eve, told me Truss's office recommended a fifth dose at night. I found this amount too much for me — it kept me up all night with extreme agitation.

Still, anxious to be well, I decided to increase my dosage to five times a day. I took the extra dose at 7am instead of 10pm. By Thursday I became ''fluish,'' then really sick by Friday night. Sore throat, pounding and inflamed swollen gums, earache, headache — close to passing out. The symptoms disappeared on Saturday then started again along with severe hunger at 1am. So I ate an entire jar of peanut butter. My chest was tightening intermittently. I also felt crazy several times, but mildly. Hot . . . . Headaches . . . . Throat very swollen and sore after 7pm dose . . . By 8pm, I felt I would pass out sitting in my rocker. It passed. I phoned Jean-Pierre long distance at 11pm, still scared. He was annoyed because I wouldn't let him rest. On top of everything, I felt a tremendous feeling of letdown. Lonely, afraid . . . shattering mentally . . . . Now I can see I was re-experiencing all my symptoms at once in a milder form. The nystatin was definitely working. (If all this seems a bit out of synch here — it is — so you can imagine how discombobulated I was writing this).

Eve had taught me many things. Alfalfa for faintness, parsley for chlorophyll and cleaning out toxins, garlic for B vitamins (B_6 for estrogen) and a natural antibiotic. Naturally grown healers — herbs and plants — I could tolerate well. She also taught me how to clean out the bloodstream with them after candida died off so the toxins wouldn't be reabsorbed into my system. And of course, 8 to 10 glasses of water per day as a minimum to flush the system. I listened and followed her directions.

When I visited Cort on March 17, he was elated and surprised. ''I've seen no one turn around like this on so small a dose of nystatin.'' He commented. ''Whatever you're doing, keep doing it.'' I did. I kept calling Eve.

He also stated three things that had happened:
   a) the organisms were dead
   b) dead and controlled
   c) my body would become resistant to the nystatin and I'd need
      to increase the dosage

''Too low,'' Cort went on, ''symptoms return. Too high, candida dies off too fast and severe flu symptoms appear plus optical neuritis and pain in joints. Recovery would be like a tooth-edged saw — up and down.''

Upon my return from Cort's office, I sat down limply and cried then phoned Jean-Pierre, Zena (my therapist in L.A.), and several friends to tell them I was returning to health, that I was on my way. Tears of joy flowed from my heart.

Difficult, adjusting to getting out of jail and death. My mind said *go-go-go* because I felt so well; my body said *no-no-no*, time to rest and recuperate. One must be finely tuned to oneself at this critical phase, for physical recovery tends to be slower than the mental. The trick at this point is to listen to one's heart because nystatin, as it heals more and more, tends to hype up the immune system with false energy. Getting support from others who have been there is very helpful when this happens; it's part of the healing. Vaguely, I recall (and this doesn't happen to everyone) a hyper-activity of my sex drive — an abnormal need for massive amounts of sex. Sounds randy, but it was just plain physically and emotionally painful. With this unusual development, Cort suggested I cut the dose for awhile. This was a blessing and a curse for candidiasis had robbed me of my sex drive; now it was overdoing it. I wept gratefully when I realized that this too was returning. I knew now I would be well.

At three weeks on nystatin I was able to be in the same room with print for an hour to begin my income tax. A monumental undertaking with my toxicity to the formaldehyde and chemicals in ink. No longer did I see one paragraph faded, the next jet black; no longer did I smell all chemicals in every product one hundred times normal. *I was healing!* Hope sprung anew in me each day as I was physically able to do more and more. The ''print room'', as I called my dining room — cum — business office, became the daily testing ground for my progress. Some days, I had chest pain, electricity pulsing up my left arm and cerebrals; others nothing.

I played a little basketball with my girls which they loved. Afterwards my jaw and head were tightening. All normal, reassured Dr. Cort when I phoned him. That evening, Joan, another E.I. sufferer, called me, miserable with cerebral suicidal depressions from mold. I empathized with her for they are the worst to survive, aside from the insanity whereby voices are screaming in your head, telling you something is going to get you. I attempted to comfort her but I don't know how much I helped. Luckily for her, my head was clear.

Let me mention here, dairy products remained *verboten*. The steamed food grew monotonous, so I called Dr. Erlander. He suggested a chemically--free olive oil now that my hydrocarbon load was lessened. He also taught me how to make ''ghee'' butter, a preparation devoid of dairy. Here's how:

1. Melt 4 sticks of butter slowly in a stainless steel or corning ware pan.
2. Place in bowl, put in refrigerator and allow to harden.
3. Scrape off the cream on top and the cheesy product on the bottom.

Now it's ready to eat. With Stig's helpful advice, I was able to add two more foods to my life.

Jean-Pierre had given me a tape of ''Evita'' for a Christmas present, which I'd been unable to play. I listened to it, then watched a T.V. film about a couple who'd been picked up by UFO's. Afterwards, all I could do was cry and cry — tears that I was getting better, joy at regaining ordinary, everyday abilities that I had lost. It was a humbling experience.

Tremendous bursts of energy shot through me. A very creative stage began. I wrote two short stories and began a satirical book on raising children, an upper-class Erma Bombeck's version. Another blessing — my children were also able to be in the same room with me without any repercussions physically. First time in 5 months.

Eve moved out of her house sporadically, avoiding the weekly spraying of malathion near her home, by which she was severely affected. Losing her assistance most of the week was difficult but I had enough information to keep me going.

Math came back! What had become impossible — adding and subtracting — from brain toxicity was not only restored but the length of time I could function increased from a few minutes to 1½ hours. To me this was a miracle!

By March 26, I was severely hyperactive. Too much nystatin? The foul green stools and abdominal bloating occurred every 3 to 4 days and were now commonplace. But it passed. Dr. Cort explained this was either too much nystatin or the immune system coming back.

On March 31, I tried to have Sr. Catherine, the high school principal, speak to me in my home concerning Jen's entering the Oakland school in the Fall. When the nun brought out newly printed material for school, I experienced chest pain, felt peculiar, heart pounding at about 140 beats, dizzy, and weakness with mental confusion. I ended the interview feeling very weak. *Resembled sugar withdrawal.* I remembered I'd been a bad girl — I ate croissants on Sunday. It caused me to re-experience all my symptoms for one hour. No more sugar! I told myself — for now.

The next day I had my hairdresser come over to cut all our hair, mine for the first time in one year. I reacted with chest pain and pain in my left arm when he entered the room. Newly dry cleaned clothes! He'd been prepared for this illness by me but misunderstood what ''clean'' meant. Willingly he put on an old cotton T-shirt and I was fine.

The hyperactivity continued on the 5 doses. Yet I was exhausted each day. Eve said this would occur as the yeast died off but to go slowly for my body hadn't caught up with the die-off. Her warm advice really soothed me. Here I noticed something else: since I started nystatin, my sensitivity to mold foods had increased. (This side effect lasts as long as one takes the drug.) Eve experienced increased sensitivity to the slightest mold in her house. Somehow I was spared.

My next "fix" or addictive food became dried green peas. Added to peanuts and carrots, I had some pleasure in life.

The next visit to Dr. Cort on March 31, he told me I had a liver enzyme, glutathione, that should be elevated in my case being a recovering alcoholic, but was totally missing. This puzzled him. Eve knew the answer. She told me this enzyme was destroyed in hydrocarbon poisoning.

She also told me that according to Dr. Truss, a Japanese study showed that sugar, in the presence of candida albicans, breaks down into ethyl alcohol. To the doctors, this fact didn't mean much. To me, a recovering alcoholic, it explained why my reactions were so severe. A drop of alcohol in a recovering alcoholic's body starts up the disease again where they left off. Even a slight amount of ethyl alcohol in my body produced "drinking symptoms." Carbohydrates "feed" the yeast; sugar is the end product of alcohol in the body.

The Japanese had been studying candidiasis since the 50's, shortly after the A-bomb was dropped on Hiroshima. It was called "mei-tei" or drinking man's disease as characterized by the pseudo-alcoholic symptoms. The Japanese knew candidiasis (caused by yeast or candida albicans) was a direct result of hydrocarbon poisoning from the radioactive fallout of the bomb.

With this bit of news to digest, Eve then referred me back to Dr. Steve Levine, the biochemist who'd had E.I., for a more technical explanation of the missing enzyme. Steve expounded, "The absence of glutathione is a complete breakdown of the oxidation system of the body which is necessary to its ability to eliminate toxins. When one loses this ability, Vitamin C supplementation and bicarbonates are converted into poisons in the liver." *That explained my severe "allergic" reaction to these compounds.* (Presently, it is believed vitamin C, along with A and E, are the chief anti-oxidants of the body.) "That's okay," he reassured me, "if you can't take anything. I'm preparing an anti-oxidant formula with glutathione which should be on the market shortly. Keep taking nystatin and this ability will return." Thanks Steve, I'm truly grateful.

Wild sexuality persistently accompanied the over-activity. Not pleasant, believe me, but rather a maddening condition. At night I was wide awake and pacing. Angry. Agitated. Eve said too much nystatin — cut down.

Jean-Pierre took a new job in Southern California near Laguna Beach which is another hour's drive south of L.A. from where he lived. It shoved a new wedge between us. One day, I would let him go. Right now, this new emotional stress added to my symptoms.

At last it dawned on me — I was having "drinking" symptoms — nervousness, anxiety, agitation, rage, cruel and negative thinking. All along I'd thought this was *me*, but it was *candida*! What a relief, after the torture I'd gone through most of my 20's and 30's, thinking "this" was me rather than multiple chemical sensitivities. I cried again with joy.

Today doctors know alcoholism and candida are connected. The alcoholic they suspect has candida manifests mercurial mood swings combined with homicidal rage and violent feelings which they may or may not act out. If the candida goes untreated, the recovering alcoholic will experience the same symptoms from chemical exposure or eating foods, particularly grains and sugar. To this very day, I avoid sugar completely and eat grains only occasionally. (This will not necessarily be true for a non-alcoholic.) In my experience working with myself and candida sufferers, sugar is the common food to be relinquished for life or the symptoms start up again.

Five weeks into nystatin therapy I was able to wash my hair with an aloe vera shampoo as recommended by Dr. Cort's office. A slight reaction — reddening — cropped up on my temples. Surely I'd come a long way in a short period of time. For washing my hair with anything at all was impossible from October til December of '81 when I discovered Erlander's homemade olive oil soap. At that point in time, I dissolved bars of his soap in a glass jar filled with bottled water allowing it to melt to its liquid form. The homemade shampoo enabled me to wash my hair from December thru April. The aloe vera shampoo breakthrough was monumental for all commercial shampoo had produced anaphylaxis up til then.

It is important to mention here that I had hired help to care for me physically throughout this whole period (Berkeley had a marvelous source of compassionate aides). Basically, I was totally dependent physically on others for I was unable to drive for a year due to car fumes causing anaphylaxis, or shop for myself, or care for my home and children. At the small Catholic school the girls were attending, another source of occasional help was provided through the priests. I needed help all the time for the generalized weakness, mixed between occasional spurts of hyperactivity, to get me through each day. I stress the need for candidiasis sufferers to have all the help they can muster, for E.I. is a disease of exhaustion, leaving the victim a very vulnerable, helpless soul. Without the assistance of a lovely woman named Vera, I wouldn't have made it.

Again, I called Cort about the severe hypersexuality. He theorized the ovaries were coming alive again. Well, that was interesting, for my periods had been reduced to a drop during the breakdown and were presently returning to normal. I suspected the entire endocrine system was coming alive, based on the hyperactivity, usually a thyroid function.

Determining what is causing reactions — the air, something you ate or drank, or clothing, so you can remove or avoid it — can bring one to the verge of true insanity. For instance, I had Vera try an unscented oil on me during a massage, convinced I was quite well. Within minutes, I had anger, agitation, and violent thinking. I washed it off and changed my clothes but some must have been absorbed because I spent the better part of the day in a miserable cerebral reaction.

On April 5, I postulated, my symptoms were returning. Time I thought to go up on the dose. Let me explain here that in early '82, very little was known about nystatin, and the daring physicians who used it knew little also. It was really up to you to take charge of your own disease.

The mold in the air was heavy again that night which created more suicidal depressions. ''Something'' told me to turn on the heater. That's how I discovered heat will penetrate the mold around you, and stop the reaction! So will showers which wash off the excessive positive ions.

On April 8, I increased my night dosage to gr $\frac{1}{16}$. Here, I started going up and feeling fine one day, then leaden and sick the following day. Somehow, I drove thirty miles away to visit an herbalist, Peko Sawa, who Eve recommended had helped her. Peko used iridology — something new to me — to determine my state of health. I was so ill at this time that she interviewed me in the street for I could not go into the toxic house she was working out of. She told me every organ in my body was severely diseased. After recommending many herbs, none of which I could touch, due to my severely debilitated condition, I went home where I slipped into a black depression. Fighting to go on again, I phoned Eve. Simultaneously, I felt drunk and disoriented. Eve commented, ''I've never heard you so bad.'' She confided to me that her friend, Anna, had gone to Dr. Truss in Alabama and reported that recovery at our stage, was years! I wrote a letter to Dr. Truss that night, outlining my case and asking his advice.

I'd spent the previous weekend at a fellow sufferer's home in West Marin without ill effects. The fellow drove to Berkeley and picked me up as I was unable to drive there myself. The trip helped my morale immensely. When I returned, full of confidence, I decided to experiment and take nystatin only 2½ hours apart at 10 and 12:30pm. By 3pm, my body felt like lead. I could barely talk or move. I remained this way for thirty minutes. The rest of the day, I was bursting with energy, even cleaning up black mold on Amy's mattress, and a wall in Jen's closet.*Nothing happened.* What success after spending the weekend in Marin!

I phoned Eve with the good news; she was delighted. She also hung on the line while I attempted to use half a nystatin suppository for the vaginitis. *Nothing happened.* The vaginal monilia was now treatable.

THE HEALING CRISIS

A healing crisis occurs when a person has been detoxifying for a certain period of time. The body begins a massive dumping of toxins which is followed by feeling great, as opposed to a sickness crisis, whereby one becomes ill then drained afterwards. It's the body's natural way of healing itself. Doctors are not familiar with this. But Eve was, for she learned from Peko. The first healing crisis occurs naturally around two months on nystatin.

With candidiasis, however, a healing crisis can be precipitated by eating a forbidden food. Millet bread proved irresistible to me. Millet, yeast, honey, and nuts — I ate the whole loaf. And vomited an hour later.

Prior to this indulgence, from April 5 to May 3, I'd slowly increased my dosage to gr 1/16, four times a day, one additional dose per week. ''If no side effect,'' Eve advised, ''continue to increase the next dose at the same time interval.'' (Going up on the dosage of nystatin too fast can also induce vomiting, nausea and severe migraines.) I followed her advice religiously. During this period I experienced severe intermittent exhaustion and spaciness. Virtually, I was non-functioning. Menses returned heavily — a new progression, after spotting periods for nearly three years.

The craving for nuts during this period was maddening. It seems candida sufferers, when exposed to chemicals or yeast die-off, universally crave nuts. My ''peanut research'' taught me that nuts contain all the essential amino-acids, calcium, niacin, and B vitamins. The nuts calm down the reaction. Unfortunately peanuts are considered very toxic. Never mind — I ate them anyway. It was the only thing that stopped the cravings. Many times one will get sick, but what else is there? I had no answers. So what did I do — continued to stuff on nuts! Now I was beginning to gain weight. That was a good sign!

Let me digress here for a moment on the peanut connection. There is a paradox in this disease. When there is a chemical exposure, such as fog, smog, or Santa Anas, which produce positive ions (body destroyers) in the air, the candida flares up. At the same time, nystatin also produces heightened chemical reactions. The patient seems to compensate for these labile, hypoglycemic reactions induced by these factors by stuffing on large amounts of nuts. Physical relief from the maddening food cravings is a catch-22: the forbidden food is the only way to calm the body.

Tryptophan, an essential amino acid and natural body tranquilizer found in nuts affects the brain as a catalyst for endorphins. Endorphins are the natural morphine of the body, producing relaxation. The candida sufferer has a breakdown in this transmission or, it is presently believed, an inability to utilize tryptophan through normal means; no one knows for sure yet. Peanuts solve the problem.

Some E.I.'s crave cashews, others peanuts or almonds. In any event, I must warn you that raw nuts are a tremendous strain on the adrenals producing more bodily stress. They are also retained in the intestinal rugae, only to sit there and ferment over time, adding to the yeast's nourishment. Therefore, I suggest roasted only. Eve also discovered placing nuts in the freezer kills the mold, thereby allowing another food into one's diet without causing a reaction or becoming ill.

There are many tricks to survival if you cannot stop eating nuts as I couldn't. In fact, the stools produced after a nut binge will help clinch the diagnosis, for a candida sufferer will produce peanut butter-consistency bowel movement. *We are our own peanut-grinding machine.* This is how moldy stools appear — grossly abnormal.

My healing crisis of May 3, began without my knowing it. Here are my notes taken from my journal:

> Exhausted ... Legs leaden ... Feel they're going to explode ... Could barely move all day ... got worse as day went on ... Feeling more and more detached ... Legs worse. Went to bed ... rolled from side to side ... Feeling left for two hours then returned and moved to my trunk — burning sensation ... ''ground glass'' in my intestines ... Head burning like acetylene torch. Thought I'd die. Then madness set in. I wanted to bash my brains out on a wall or die. Rolled from side to side on my green-frame bed, screaming to God for release from this madness. Just like withdrawal from alcohol 2½ years ago. It comes in waves. Head full of despair, fear and paranoia — the toughest. Urge to jump out window to stop voices ... Overwhelming ... Jean-Pierre and Zena talked to me by phone ... Couldn't hear them — I was insane, detached, feared I'd end my life ... Fell into an exhausted sleep at 2am.

The rest of the crisis was recorded in retrospect a week later. The only way I could recall what happened at all was to re-run the story backwards from Sunday to the previous Monday when it all began. Here is the rest of the drama.

Tuesday - I have too vague a memory. Only remember a nurse's aide showing up. Too ill and exhausted to show her anything. Stopped the nystatin completely and restarted 10pm on Wednesday.

Wednesday, May 5, I felt worse and worse. By 10am I felt I was dying. Called Dr. Cort — go to the local Emergency Room for CBC, UA and poisoning tests. Exhausted, almost losing consciousness on and off. Emotional strain and fear horrible. At the hospital I stayed outside because I smelled heavy perfume as I opened the door, fearing my body couldn't withstand any more. A nurse, similar to Nurse Ratchitt in "One Flew Over The Cuckoo's Nest," refused to help me. I laid down on the ground outside whilst being interviewed by a kindly young male clerk. As they were about to take me in, three ambulances arrived and I was tabled. I called Cort's office from a payphone, told his receptionist I was collapsing outside the hospital and they were too busy to see me. (Guess I didn't look gray enough.) Screamed at Cort's office help "I'll go home" when they wouldn't put him on the phone. I lay on the street outside the parking garage, waiting for my aide to bring the car. My breathing was labored and I couldn't stand up. Cort must have done something, for Nurse "Ratchitt" came outside, calling my name. I crawled across the street back to the hospital totally dazed. She took my vital signs on a chair in the hallway. Then she drew blood. My breathing was very labored. Finally, they put me on a table where a doctor checked me. He said my breathing was abnormal — hyperventilation. I said it was the disease. Per usual they treated me for stress. Well, I sure was! They placed me in observation for several hours. The air conditioning and oxygen helped. Despite all this, it turned out well. *I lived!* Doctor said I was having an "anxiety attack." I screamed at him, "This was the result of rapid kill off of toxins." He patted me patronizingly on the head, refusing to bother Cort with the results. Went home and felt better for a few hours. Nose and head became severely stuffed. Felt severely detached ... in dream world. Fear ... Paranoia ... Wanted to kill myself to stop voices in my head. Called Cort again ... Felt I should be hospitalized — given cortisone. Christ no, I'm a recovering alcoholic, I'll go more insane. I refused his advice. Called Jean-Pierre. Said he'd be up on next plane (45-minute flight). Madeleine (an aide) sat with me as I rolled back and forth on my bed with the madness, telling her I couldn't take any more. "It" subsided around 8 or 9pm. Jean-Pierre arrived a little after

10pm. Fear, crying, paranoia til 3am as he held me. Felt better Thursday morning although weak and tired. Jean-Pierre cared for me all day. I couldn't move my head for my brain seemed bruised. I had to hold my head with both hands or the blood rushed to my crown and the pain was excruciating. Jean-Pierre left at 10pm. Cort had warned me not to start the nystatin again, but I was experiencing withdrawal symptoms from the drug. Cort was so concerned, he called Dr. Truss in Alabama. He didn't know what to do either, not having seen a case this severe. Basically I had relived *delirium tremens* and then some.

Thursday is a complete blank.

Friday was the first clear day all week — felt wonderful for a few hours then sick and exhausted. Dr. Cort called again. I told him about the horror story I'd been living the past three days. He commented he'd not seen anyone that sick but he seemed to listen. Later on that day, as I stayed on my minimum dosage (gr $\frac{1}{32}$ - four times a day), ''the headache'' began — different from yesterday's vise-like head pain. Now there was pressure and pain through my left eye.

Looking back at this now, it's amazing I had any clarity at all to record anything! Fuzzily, I remembered Dr. Cort mentioning Herxheimer's reaction.

''Wow, you're having Herxheimer's reaction,'' he said. ''That's what happened to syphilitics back in the 20's and 30's when they were treated with arsenicals. What happens,'' he went on, ''is the candida organism dies off from the nystatin producing approximately seventy toxins. The toxins then pour into the blood stream causing a crisis. If the yeast die-off is too fast, the reaction the person experiences is an acute poisoning. Be careful Elizabeth,'' he warned, ''We don't want this to happen again. You were on too much nystatin for your body. Stay on a minimal dosage.''

Let me reassure you my healing crisis was not the usual. Most people in earlier stages experience severe flu-like symptoms for 4 to 5 days when taking nystatin. But the people recovering from alcohol and/or drug abuse must go especially slowly on nystatin to prevent what happened to me. I went up on the dose too rapidly, working with a very unknown factor, in my desire to get well too fast. There is no getting well fast at this extreme level of candidiasis. It is a slow, rocky, roller-coaster recovery. But you do become functioning again. I did.

Very few people have my experience. Yet I urge you, if you choose this course of treatment to proceed very slowly. There are alternatives to nystatin, which I will discuss later on in this book. Patience is a necessary virtue all candidiasis sufferers must learn.

Now I knew why Eve was so concerned. She knew of this danger and was greatly relieved to hear I was still alive. Without her tutelage, I doubt that I would have gone on with the drug. But it was nystatin or a slow death. Truly, I was blessed by her mentress-ship.

After "losing" nearly two weeks out of my life, I was thrilled to go out on Mother's Day. It fell on May 10th. Fearfulness of everything was now added to my physical symptoms from my seven months of isolation. Unlike agoraphobia, the fears were based on real, life-threatening reactions to chemicals.

Yet there is a humorous side to this horror. For going outside into the world is always an adventure. Having someone with you aware of your limitations can be very helpful. For instance, Jean-Pierre accompanied me to an "indoor" art show (Going indoors is "out" in E.I.), full of exquisite Greco-Roman deity paintings. Smoke, perfume and so on blasted me as I walked into the shop. Spaced, I signalled to Jean-Pierre with my foggy eyes; he pulled my going limp-to-unconsciousness body out the door. We'd been accustomed to these bizarre departures from most events. A laugh always followed our rehash of how strange we must look. Really, it was pretty funny.

Although exhaustion came in waves the rest of the day, I was elated that I was able to go out at all. Enjoying life really heals the physical body tremendously.

Early recovery is very tough but it does get better if you just hang in there, follow the diet, avoid severe chemical exposures (tar, paint, cigarettes etc.), and take nystatin, telling yourself over and over, "I will be well." You will.

The encouraging phase of recovery is when you begin to notice that the reaction occurs but doesn't last as long. And it is less severe as each day passes. You do not go backwards, although you may feel that way at times. Relapses — or crises — or severe exposures are limited in the damage they can do to your body once you've instituted therapy. You are on your way.

On May 18 there were more side effects from nystatin. Continuing on the low dose, gr $\frac{1}{32}$, I now experienced another frightening phenomenon. As I was sitting in my backyard, the sensation of one hundred bright yellow photographer's bulbs went off in front of my eyes, temporarily almost completely blinding me, followed by seeing hazily through a bright yellow film. Knife-like pain followed through the left side of my head. I'd also been experiencing depression, apathy, and shakes, accompanied by violent feelings. Dr. Cort told me to go off nystatin for one week. I asked him if this were optic neuritis which could lead to blindness. "Not on such low doses," he reassured me. *Not on such low doses — everything and some things they'd not heard of were happening to me on low doses.*

I followed his advice for one day, recalling the withdrawal symptoms of my last attempt. Then the shakes began along with cravings for nuts. So I went back on nystatin Thursday — using four doses of gr $\frac{1}{32}$ once again. It didn't seem enough for it did not alleviate my symptoms. But I was too frightened to take any more; I was alone during the day with the children being in school.

Going on and off nystatin in this yo-yo fashion produced severe food cravings. I stuffed on peanuts all week til the co-op store ran out of unsalted peanuts! The cravings ceased the fourth day back on the drug.

That weekend, I tried something very daring — I drove across the Oakland Bay Bridge to visit a fellow E.I. What a triumph! Five months earlier, I couldn't make it across the bridge with oxygen, car filter, and a driver. His house was very moldy which made me irritable and angry. Still, this was tremendous progress.

Returning to Berkeley wasn't good. There were lots of car fumes and smog when I drove back. Halfway across the bridge I felt spaced out and faint. By the time I reached my house, I had slurred speech, spaciness, and suicidal thinking. Crying uncontrollably, I called Jean-Pierre who was in Palo Alto visiting his children. He was very upset. ''Come back to L.A. with me.'' His offer was totally unrealistic. Due to my prolonged isolation, I could now only survive in my chemically-free house. Goodbye to him. Called Zena, my lifeline in L.A. The madness passed an hour or two after we spoke.

The past few weeks had taken their toll on me. The next three nights I slept 10-12 hours. I was going too fast again. Dr. Cort had warned me, ''You'll feel great but pace yourself or you'll have a relapse.'' I didn't listen.

On May 19, I increased nystatin again to adding a dose (gr $\frac{1}{16}$) before bedtime. Another milestone occurred that day too. Unable to take any vitamins or minerals up til this point, I experimented with whole rice B-complex which was free of yeast, sugar and fillers — no reaction. Health was on its way!

Believe it or not, a new side effect appeared from nystatin — severe left shoulder pain. Having experienced bursitis previously in my right shoulder during my 20's, I knew this pain was identical. Puzzled, I called Cort. ''Presently it is believed the immuneplexes cause this reaction.'' *No, can't be, bet it's gases given off by the toxins dying off.* Stubbornly, I kept raising the dosage slightly. For me, this was a mistake. Three and a half months on nystatin, I was able to add vitamin B_6 to my regime. Three or four hundred milligrams per day greatly relieved the severe pre-menstrual symptoms that accompany candidiasis. Each time I increased nystatin's dosage I went crazy with food cravings. Alfalfa sprouts helped somewhat, but only peanuts sated me. Bottled spring water no longer caused shock. Organic cucumbers and avocado were added to my diet without incidence.

Bravely, I attended two of my children's functions. An outdoor picnic at the ''Strawberry,'' a grassy recreational area for UC Berkeley faculty and students, was fine until barbecuing began. Numbness of my body and faintness followed. Perfume produced shakes and anger. Despite this, we were able to stay for the entire event by constantly changing where we sat.

The other outing, Amy's violin recital, was impossible for it was indoors full of perfume and aftershave. I lasted ten minutes, *but I made an appearance.* Physically being able to go anywhere around ordinary life, even for five minutes, always lifted my spirits.

By Saturday, crying and despair overtook me again. The shoulder pain became severe and unmitigated. Again, I wanted to die. Again, rolling on my green spring bed, crying out to God for help. A miracle occurred that night.

A quote from my diary of May 30, 1982 describes the incident:

Another incredible experience last night. Went to bed and prayed for God to help me. I was restless and half asleep when I had to urinate. In a daze, I sat up and looked up at my window. The blanket, which I used for a shade to cover the bathroom window, was transformed. The room was very warm and lit up with a bright white light. (The bathroom lights were not on.) On the brown blanket, the muted form of Christ appeared in ivory-white priestly robes, looking down on me. His face was unclear. His arms were spread out across the blanket; His palms turned upward. His head bowed to the right side, He "beamed" compassion into me. A compassion that flooded my very being, beyond anything one could experience on earth. A gentle voice, telepathically said "You will not die of this disease. I am with you always from now on."

Then, a heavy pressure "formed" something solid in my solar plexus area, removing totally my feelings of abandonment, despair and aloneness.

I was frightened and felt nothing was quite real, and crawled under the covers like a small child, hiding myself from the unknown.

Shakily, I decided to come out and see if what I'd seen was real. I closed my eyes and felt my way to the toilet where I sat down. Quaking with fear, I reached for the light switch and turned it on.

The blanket was a blanket. Relieved, I returned to bed and turned off the lights. I looked at the blanket again. It had the slight appearance of a person fading, but it wasn't the same as I'd seen. The room became nighttime cool. The white light was gone.

Had I been hallucinating from the nystatin or had I really seen Jesus? I decided to call Fr. Peter, my spiritual advisor, the next day, and share this happening with him.

Still shook, but very peaceful, I fell asleep.

The next day I sat in the movie "Reds" for 3½ hours (theater almost empty — not recently sprayed with pesticides), and went to Mass. Perfume didn't affect me. I was in awe.

After Mass, I visited Fr. Peter and told him my story. Unexpectedly, he said, "I believe you. You've renewed my faith in the Maker." Still perplexed by my "visitation," I shared my doubts again with him at what I'd seen.

"Just think of it this way Elizabeth. God removed people, food, clothing and everything else from you that we live with in this world. I believe there is a message. Nothing stands between you and the Maker. He wants something from you. You'd better listen." It would take me a long time to digest what had happened that night.

On May 31, I was able to go into a friend's house for fifteen minutes without reacting. A blessing. I was so grateful.

Fever blisters began breaking out all over my mouth. Heavy period. Result of tomato? Or is candida die-off related to the herpes virus?

There is a reason I am presenting such great detail at this stage of recovery, for the first few months on nystatin are the most difficult while the most physical progress also takes place. In my case, this was very dramatic on very small doses. All Cort could say was, "I don't know what you're doing but keep doing it." And so I did.

What he didn't know was Eve was my lay advisor. Her advice opened a new dimension to me in healing. Being a trained nurse, orthodox medicine was my narrow perspective. Herbs were beyond my knowledge but I was open. Through her guidance, more and more doors opened to me in my healing. The diet, the vitamins, the parsley — all were working well.

That's why I've been so painstaking in my details, for I want you to know you are not alone, that more and more is added back into your life each day and it's a slow process.

Eve taught me to add only one new herb or vitamin at a time then wait a week to see what happens. The same holds true for foods and increasing the dose of nystatin. In this way, it will be clearer exactly what is affecting you. I gladly pass this wisdom on to you.

Most failures to recover from candidiasis are from an unwillingness to change and do what is necessary to get well. In speaking with these people who tell me they cannot take nystatin I find several things are consistent:

a) they are not following the diet.
b) they took too large a dose to begin with and were frightened off.
c) they are still exposing themselves daily to major chemicals.
d) they are still wearing synthetic clothing, nail polish, hair spray, or cosmetics.

If one wants to recover from this critical phase, I found it's imperative to follow the regimen, remembering it is not forever. One day you will be back in the real world. Just keep trucking.

Right around May, I ended my relationship with Jean-Pierre. His priorities being himself and staying married preyed on my mind in an abnormal way. Sickness makes everything out of proportion, but negative stress contributes greatly to the detaining of one's recovery. The man was confused. Did I need this — no. So I let him go — for now.

Obstinately, I continued on the higher dose of gr $\frac{1}{16}$ despite miserable cerebrals and shoulder pain. Determined to get well, I said to myself, *let's get on with it.*

My plan was shattered shortly thereafter. On June 20, a vandal spray painted my car. Angrily, I jumped into the car, late for a dental appointment for Amy. Suddenly, I could barely breathe. Severe pain struck my right lung.

The sound of fluid gushed through my lungs as I collapsed over the wheel of my car. *This is it.* I told myself, terrified.

Somehow I made it back to the house. My color was gray. Began losing consciousness. Feeling of dying. Crawled to phone, dialed Eve. ''Elizabeth, I know you're afraid, but I gave this to a friend of mine with our disease who I found just as she was going to hang herself from a tree in a severe cerebral. And it pulled her out of it.'' She was referring to immuno-glandplex. This new development would be another major turning point in my recovery. For immunplex is a glandular, non-toxic immune system compound, devised by biochemist Dr. Steven Levine, to balance the immune system — bring it up if it were too low; pull it down if it were hyperactive.

Everything was going dim. Barely conscious, I asked Amy to bring me an immunplex. I'd tried one previously — shock was the result. Adrenalin was in my purse. Phenol would kill me in my present condition. Immunplex or death.

Clinging to Eve by phone was my lifeline as I, petrified, placed half of the contents of the beef gelatin capsule in my mouth. We were taking no chances I'd react on the capsule itself. Just about holding ''our'' breath, I swallowed it. Within minutes, it worked! My brain cleared up. The chest pain was alleviated. Thank God! For vasculitis (arterial spasm) is life-threatening by closing off the blood flow to that side of your body. Half of me was blue-gray, the other waxen. I'd say my condition was grave.

We were both so relieved, I began crying. This was an awesome responsibility Eve had undertaken. I blessed her again. Then I took a second one and *all* the symptoms disappeared. Only to return an hour later. In between capsules, I phoned Steve to ask how many I could take safely in one day. ''Eight,'' he said, ''with tons of water. Try the Vitamin C powder too Elizabeth.'' By now I'd try anything that would help.

For sure, I was set back. My body reacted on everything just as it had at my sickest eight months earlier. *No, God, please don't let me stay this way, I begged — I couldn't bear it again.*

For three days I went up and down. The vitamin C powder caused nausea, vomiting and collapse. Telephoned Steve again. He suggested another supplement. ''Go carefully on the amino acids if your liver is compromised.'' Mine was. I couldn't physically tolerate his formula — I went into shock placing a pinhead amount on my tongue. ''Stop the C — you're toxic to it.'' Likewise, the amino acids.

Back to talking by phone, covered by a cotton blanket in order not to induce more chest pain from the plastic. Off nystatin again. Dr. Cort said one word when I phoned — ''Jesus — that's horrible.'' (Whenever you have a heavy chemical exposure, you cut back on nystatin for your body will start reacting on that chemical too.) ''Call me anytime,'' he said.

Miraculously, the setback lasted only one week. When I called Steve to let him know how I was doing, I told him I had a slight headache and severe diarrhea the past few days. (This is not ordinary diarrhea but one loses pints of water rectally at rapid intervals, then collapses.) ''Wow,'' he exclaimed ''You must have had some poisoning!'' I certainly did.

This episode left me completely exhausted for several weeks. Summer was upon me. Intuitively, I knew I would not survive the summer if I didn't send my girls elsewhere to be taken care of; in my serious condition the normal stress of two young girls would have killed me. Plans were made to send them to camp for one month, then to my sister Dee in New York for August. Their cousins, girls the same ages, were thrilled. I was relieved, for I also knew that two months of being alone with the aid of Vera, would produce a great deal of healing. I was right.

June 26. I was sitting packing Amy's clothing for camp when my elbows turned bright red and burned up followed by huge blotches on my ears, knees, neck and shoulders. Everything frightened me now. With each new reaction my only thought was, when will anaphylaxis hit overload and my life be all over? Scared out of my mind, I called Eve as my head raced back over all my textbook knowledge of anaphylaxis I'd learned, plus my personal experiences in the Emergency Room. I knew it was fast and fatal without adrenalin as an antidote, which the doctors were afraid to give me.

After all these episodes of suffering so much, I finally realized that gr $\frac{1}{32}$ four times a day was my dose for healing and not a smidgen more. A semi-stability entered my life for a short while.

Filters can be a very important part of recovery. A friend with E.I. said she'd found a new filter that purified and ionized the air in one's house. She brought it over for Joseph Mann and me to test out, for if anyone would react, we would since both of us were so sick.

The air produced smelled mountainous. We both liked it. I felt slightly agitated but ignored this for I never knew what else was causing the reaction.

Another episode of burning redness occurred at this time. My liquid soap? Mystery is a great part of this disease. In the interim, I ''lost'' my car for six weeks waiting for the paint to ''gas'' out. Another E.I. woman told me there was a special sealer, non-toxic, which her husband used on other candidiasis people's cars. Getting my car to him in Hayward was a monu-mental task considering I could not leave my home, rent a car, take a cab or the pony express. *Forced to purchase another car!* Fortunately an E.I. lady moving back to Germany, sold me her toxin-free car. Providence shone on me that day.

Joseph called one night terrified, saying ''My heart and pulse are over 140. My brain is insane — help me. Planes are going overhead to San Francisco airport and sound as if they're inside my head.''

''Turn off the new filter'' I said gently.

''What?''

''Turn off the new filter. I discovered I was getting like that. They must have used chemicals to produce the 'mountain air' odor rather than the natural effect they claimed.''

He did as I told him. ''My God,'' he said, ''You're right. All my symptoms are gone.''

So much for the new filter we'd found!

Sherry Thomson, my Berkeley therapist with E.I., came over to my house to muscle test me for vitamins and minerals I wanted to try. Muscle testing is an innocuous method used to test the body's reaction without putting the substance into one's body, thereby causing further harm. It is done by having the person put her strongest arm straight out in front of the body. The other person places one hand on the forehead; with the other hand she tries to press the wrist down while the person resists. You place the substance against your heart. This simple procedure will teach the person tested if she is allergic to a new substance. If the arm cannot be pushed down, it's all right to try it; if the arm weakens and is easily pushed downwards, the substance will have an adverse affect. Safe and simple. Many people have been protected from unnecessary suffering by this procedure.

Skeptical though I was, almost believing this modern day witchcraft, I had Sherry test me for sea minerals (O.K.) amino acids (shocky), so I added Nutricology's allergy formula II (sea minerals) to my retinue. Combined with the immunplex, more protection is provided against chemicals. Sea minerals are comprised of natural selenium, iodine, and kelp.

This was a boon to my system to start building it up again. Vitamin E is necessary to utilize selenium but I was unable to tolerate it yet. Perhaps a little would be absorbed? Steve's amino acids have helped pull many people out of reactions but were contraindicated in my case. The immunplex helps strengthen the immune system, for I found it was the foundation for me to be able to add many other nutrients.

There's a peculiar effect with this disease. As you heal, you don't realize it consciously. Usually a family member or friend will say, ''Hey, you didn't react on that!'' The healing becomes subtle at this point. Like green stools just disappeared one day, in my fourth month on nystatin.

The turning blotchy bright red, still puzzled me. Was it the orange rug I touched, the bottled water? Didn't know. I tried distilled water again. Surely that was it.

Jean-Pierre was destined to come into my life again. After two months apart, I phoned him. He was happy to hear from me. Said he enjoyed being alone doing what he wanted. Hated him and invited him up for Fourth of July weekend. He accepted happily.

Believe me, I was glad to have him back in more ways than one — for I needed him physically, mentally, and spiritually. Physically especially, as the owners of the house I was renting from phoned in June to tell me they were moving back in at Christmas. Move! Why I could barely leave my home! What to do? An inner voice said *move back to your own home in Santa Monica.* But I thought — smogsville U.S.A. — that's crazy!

Seeing Jean-Pierre again fulfilled many needs. First of all, I received lots of loving. But more importantly, I moved back into my bedroom. That can be credited to barrier cloth, a close-weaved, cotton covering which slides over the mattress like a plastic mattress cover, zips and, theoretically, seals in all the toxic fumes. It worked — for I was able to sleep in a bed for the first time in six months. This was heaven on earth. I needed Jean-Pierre to put the barrier cloth on my bed.

Jean-Pierre loves to travel. After spending a day getting reacquainted, he drove me to Santa Cruz, a resort town on the Pacific Ocean two hours south of San Francisco, to find me a cleaner environment than Berkeley. The Berkeley Hills where I lived were downwind of Richmond's refineries ten miles away and northeast of heavy chemical plant pollutions. Besides all this, the heavy fog eight months out of the year (November through June), combined with all San Francisco's pollution blown there by the ocean winds, produced a chemical nightmare where E.I.'s tended to be the sickest.

Our trip to Santa Cruz was beautiful with the exception of headache and nausea passing Montara and El Granada, heavy mold areas by the Pacific Ocean. The drive itself was nourishing. The town was clean. More than I expected, a lot more — a cross between Santa Barabara, Palm Springs and La Jolla. Peaceful. Windy areas on the west; hot and muggy on the east. For a while I felt well there, then started collapsing and feeling exhausted. The elation over the trip overshadowed my judgment. I ignored how I felt, writing it off as the stress — even good stress of getting out and going somewhere. I was wrong.

The next plan was to attempt to fly to Santa Monica in August, and spend a week in my home, while my tenants were away on a three month trip. Absolutely terrified of traveling now, since I knew why I felt so badly in planes — pesticides, formaldehyde, cigarette smoke and hydrocarbon laden people. People, places and things had become the enemy. The 20th Century could not support my life. I was like an alien from outer space. E.I. friends suggested I move to Mt. Shasta. A colony of people with this disease had moved into this isolated mountain region, a six-hour drive above San Francisco. Most of those who went to Shasta were early cases who went through ''ecology units'' to be detoxified from the 20th Century.

Ecology units are spartan, sterile, chemically-free, experimental hospital units where even the nurses and doctors must wash in baking soda before entering so as not to cause severe reactions in the patients. The theory is to remove everything that is making the person ill — approximately 2000 hydrocarbons in food, water, clothing and air.

Many doctors also suggest moving to a ''clean'' environment. In my own personal experience, physically moving away from everything and everybody you know to a remote area is more devastating than staying in a polluted area and healing there. In my research of places to live, I have not found anywhere in this country that doesn't have something toxic. Fellow E.I.'s report their experiences to me from around the nation.

One friend moved to New York City — sulfur fumes proved her undoing. Another fled to Las Vegas — felled by phenol fumes in the air. A third went to San Francisco and had suicidal depressions when the fog rolled in.

The point being — moving with this disease is not an answer. I lived in heavily polluted Berkeley and began to get better. *It's an inside job — the willingness to take action and do the necessary physical steps to heal.* By this I do not mean this disease is mental. *It is not.* However, the mental and physical symptoms to me are a manifestation of a soul sickness permeating our society in general — toxic living. Henceforth, the ''inside job'' is changing one's attitude while simultaneously changing one's outside life.

Hence it was Santa Cruz or Santa Monica for me. Berkeley was out. No point moving into another house in this area — I wanted out of there. It goes without saying how much added stress this was for I had to move my children again. This would be our third move in four years.

After Jean-Pierre left I discovered little vesicles on my genital labia. Herpes? Oh God! Only Jean-Pierre could have brought that to me. Believe it or not, I was too ill to connect the two. Now I had herpes to worry about. When I phoned Jean-Pierre he denied any other contact. Then he told me he was planning on moving to Newport Beach for his job (an hour south of Santa Monica — seems he kept moving further south away from me). And to Paris for Christmas for three weeks. This on top of everything else was too much. I raved at him. Where do I fit into your life? Nowhere, I said. He seemed to have a knack for making a bad situation worse. Sadly enough for me, I still needed him. So I dumped him anyway.

July 1, I paid another visit to Dr. Cort. Drove the bridge myself with an emergency driver along. I did fine. Ray said my blood tests were improved. He felt Santa Cruz would be a good move for me as many E.I.'s had done very well there. Joyfully I told him I could tolerate minerals. ''Great — every time you can use supplements to build up your body, you've made another giant step forward.'' I always felt better after seeing Cort's optimistic persona — except when he'd washed his hands with scented soap before entering the room, causing me to collapse. ''Nystatin,'' I told him, ''causes severe neck and left shoulder pain if the dose is too high. When I reduce the dosage slightly the pain disappears within 3 to 4 days.'' He thanked me for sharing my experience, for so little was really known about long-term side effects of nystatin being administered in massive doses. We had already learned together that as the candida continued dying off slowly, more and more foods and supplements could be added, thereby accelerating the healing. Vitamin C was still a no-no in any form for me. Hope rang in my brain as I smilingly drove back to Berkeley.

The mystery of the bright red blotching still plagued me. I'd changed my water from spring to distilled and back again. No change. I suspected exposure to print. I became light sensitive again — also blinded by lights. Was it nystatin, print, or water causing this? It frightened me, but went away when I took an immunplex. Shortly, there would be an answer.

Eve had told me long before, in some vague memory, that the healing of this disease would be like running every illness you ever had backwards until you reached childhood. And then you were well! This important piece of information proved beneficial over and over again, as I relived my life's old physical injuries and infections. She gave me a large dose of hope that I was healing instead of getting sick again.

No matter how many times I attempted to raise the dose above gr $\frac{1}{32}$ four times a day, I met with failure. The side effects were so severe, that I knew my gr $\frac{1}{32}$ was a less sensitive person's gr $\frac{1}{2}$. This was finally settled — my body had determined a healing dose.

Between July 10 and my move to Santa Monica, I experienced more of the same roller-coaster healing. Exposed to barbecue smoke, I collapsed; immunplex pulled me out. Moderate pain in right knee. Hmm, old symptom of rheumatic fever. Exposed to home perm on my nurse's aid — anger and rage. Up on nystatin again, down when shoulder pain appeared.

One more journey was made to Santa Cruz. A fellow E.I. let me stay for three days to see if I could survive there. Temperature 98°, humidity 99%. All the cerebrals returned by dusk — fear, paranoia, voices coming to get me, crying and depression. At night, when the fog rolled in, my color became waxen, my nail beds blue. *God, I can barely breathe.* Respirations were shallow all night.

The subsequent night my condition grew worse. Voices telling me to jump off the cliffs combined with viselike chest pain. Hillary had gone out. *Terror-stricken.* Some spark of sanity reminded me to turn on the heater and her filter. Better. My trip was cut short. I fled Santa Cruz dejected.

Berkeley never looked so good — I was better there. Funny, people with advanced candidiasis go crazy in Santa Cruz, but Hillary could tolerate it. She was pretty well. Poor woman also could not travel anywhere else. Isolated. I empathized with her.

More depression, crying, insanity, exhaustion and green stools. And so it continued. A seven day healing crisis ensued from July 21 to July 28. Again, I felt better and stronger. Eve, dear Eve, didn't have the heart to tell me there would be more healing crises. Now I knew. The good news is this one was much milder than the first, and shorter. It appeared approximately two months after the first one. The pattern formed — expect a healing crisis, shorter and shorter every two months for awhile. Okay.

Thank God my girls were at camp during the month of July, for as I predicted, my body took quantum leaps in healing during this time. When they returned, I announced we were probably going back to Santa Monica in September. They were overjoyed. And then I packed them off to my sister's house in New York for August while I checked to see if I could survive in Santa Monica.

The plane ride went well. Southern California was predictable for this time of year — high heat and double smog — yet I did very well. Being with Jean-Pierre for a week helped my morale even though he seemed distant.

The best part was seeing old friends at AA. Although I could only visit with them outdoors downwind, it warmed my heart to see people who knew and cared for me. Most were shocked at my condition; none could believe I stayed sober through this ordeal; others couldn't believe I looked so healthy but was so ill. Dorian Gray turned inside out.

The decision was out of my hands. We'd return to Santa Monica — our home.

When I returned to Berkeley, Erlander's special-made cotton bed arrived. For the first five days in a row, I felt absolutely wonderful. Purchasing this expensive item had taken a great deal of research for I'd heard many E.I.'s had bought new beds or futons, then had to sell or discard them because they reacted on the toxic chemicals in the covering material. I had two companies send me samples of the cloth used in their beds for me to sleep on: one's bedding material reacted on me — pounding hands and feet; Erlander's was fine. Stig washes the material himself in his home-made washing soda, then sends it to the factory to be made into a bed. (The bed was well worth it, I do believe today: it helped relieve the hydrocarbon stress on my body.) In just five days I was able to accomplish more than I had in the past five years. The only time I felt bad physically now was when the air was humid.

Another monkey wrench was thrown my way. The DMV sent me my driver's license renewal. No way could I go into that building filled with perfume and cigarettes and take the renewal test. I had to stall for time. After several phone calls to the DMV, a supervisor told me to write to Sacramento to ask if I could renew it by mail. This bought me some time.

By the way, I discovered what caused the red blotches. Double dosing on vitamin B complex produced a niacin reaction — that's all. Simple, so simple I missed it.

As of August 16, I'd been on nystatin five and one-half months. Although I was slowly getting better, I was still severely isolated. The physical isolation from life, combined with the inability to be touched by another human being, (unless they were dressed in cotton washed in baking soda, and bathed in olive oil soap and unscented shampoo), was taking its toll. Each day became a fight to go on. I cried out to my Creator, please help me. An answer came the following day.

PAU D'ARCO

Earlier in August, I'd phoned to tell Eve I was moving to Santa Monica on September 1. She was sorry to see me go and wished me well. But she had a little secret. Peko had found a tree bark from Brazil called Pau D'arco or taheebo. The producers claimed it had been boiled into the form of a tea and used to cure cancer. Apparently, wherever this tree grew in the jungle, no fungus lived. So she thought we could try it for candida albicans, our particular fungus. Eve had been on the anti-fungal jungle tea about three weeks, and had stopped reacting on almost everything. She'd also been on nystatin for almost two years and healed just so far, like me.

Alleliua! This was music to my ears. Where can I get some? ''Phone Peko, she'll send it to you.'' I did. ''There are two kinds of taheebo,'' Eve explained, ''yellow the weakest, and purple the strongest.'' The brand she'd tried was ''A Natureza,'' a combination of the two. It was free of pesticides and all chemicals. Eve would know, for if the company had misrepresented itself, she would react adversely to it.

My prayers were answered. This could be the final healing of candidiasis. I was overjoyed. Eve promised to send me all the literature she had at present on it. Great! Great! Just great!

The anti-fungal jungle tea arrived on August 17. I went to the Berkeley pier and prayed about taking it. Is this God's answer to my prayers? I'll know shortly.

Peko included these instructions for preparation:

   1) place four cups of bottled water in stainless steel pan.
   2) sprinkle one tablespoon of taheebo bark on top of the water.
   3) bring the water to a boil on high heat.
   4) allow bark and water to boil for five minutes.
   5) remove from heat and let stand for twenty minutes.

6) strain into a glass jar or bowl removing all bark.
7) refrigerate
(Taheebo retains its potency for approximately three days).

Eve said it smelled good. Tasted a little like vanilla. I laughed and said, ''Eve, nothing we've had to take with this disease tastes good.'' I took one smell. Phew! Felt like vomiting. Should I take it or not, now that I had it? I'd become convinced it wouldn't kill me after I spoke to Eve's friend Roz S., who told me she was doing great on it too; she who had candida, from antibiotics, since she was 7 years old. At 39, she'd been a basket case before nystatin. Now she was reporting that she could stand next to barbecues and glue in one week with ''nothing happening.'' If she could do it, I could.

Out of my reverie, I stood before the nauseating taheebo. Eve was drinking four cups a day, the recommended amount. Hmm, I told myself, anything Eve does, I can do about one-quarter of. At this juncture, I'd become truly an experimenter with the totally unknown. Well, not quite. Sherry Thompson muscle-tested me — the taheebo came up pure.

I took it. Dizziness and nausea appeared after the first cup. Abdomen became very bloated after a few hours. Some abdominal pain.

August 19 was my last visit to Dr. Cort's office before I moved. I walked in and collapsed. Fresh paint in his new office. I couldn't believe it! He knew what could happen to us. After he picked me up off the floor, he wanted to give me adrenalin. No, I waved him away, semi-conscious. Threw two immunplex down my throat. A crying jag and shaking chills resulted. I recovered but exhaustion set in while my legs ached badly. More tea at 2pm. Nausea. Exhausted, rested til 10pm. Then energy, energy, energy, just as Eve said. I needed this to pack (The movers did most of it, but I decided it was time to let go of unnecessary items).

The combination of the new cotton bed and the taheebo produced a wonderful effect! The exhaustion *gone* since August 21. Now I had bundles of energy. Whooppee!! The Pau really worked! A blessing.

The second day of taheebo I had severe bloating, nausea, and nervous energy. Both days I'd felt like passing out around 5:30pm, but it only lasted half an hour.

The third day the tea was okay. Bloating decreased. Urinating large amounts. Drank the tea in small amounts all day to keep a balance in my system instead of blasting it with an entire cup. Legs aching. Exhaustion again. Walked pier for forty-five minutes. Pain in right upper quadrant of my abdomen after last dose.

By the eighth day, I felt I was well on my way to recovery. Foolishly, I believed what I read in the manual about my self-cleaning oven using only heat. I turned it on and went out. When I returned at 2pm, the house had a chemical smell. Headache, nausea, severe vertigo. Took two immunplex. Fr. Peter, my Dominican priest and friend, stopped by. As I talked to him outside, I felt better. Back in the house — severe dizziness, faint. Skipped the 3pm nystatin. I stumbled to my backyard and lay outside. *Losing consciousness lying down.* In and out of gray fog. Figured I needed food. Went in house — chest pain, dizziness. Back to the yard. Then heavy fog and mold rolled in. By now I was completely terrified. Felt the ''dying feeling'' again. Phoned Vera and Sherry: both concerned but not available to come over. Called Jean-Pierre at home in L.A. ''Don't hang up, please don't. I'm all alone and I feel like I'm dying.'' He stayed on the phone with me for an hour and held my heart as I went through trying Vitamin C and immunplex. Finally I had shaking chills, goose bumps, diarrhea and viselike right-sided chest pain.

Could this be a healing crisis? I didn't know. Too many other factors blurred my vision. I holed up in my upstairs bedroom with the electric heaters and filter. I felt better. There were toxic fumes downstairs. However they dissipated by 11pm. Feeling much better, I skipped the tea and slept exhaustedly. I decided to stop the Pau D'Arco until I was completely adjusted to my move to Santa Monica. Sherry Thompson said to expect problems physically around the third week in a new environment, for that was about the time it took for the body to start reacting on the environmental changes. There would be enough changes to deal with without attempting the Pau D'Arco on top of them. If I reacted badly to the taheebo after a while, I wouldn't know if it were the tea or the environment. I decided to wait to continue it. As little additional stress as possible with any change. Whether it be diet, drug, water or environment. At this point in time, this is the only way you can tell what is affecting you.

Fever blisters, burning gums, vaginal discharge raged the past few weeks since my visit to Jean-Pierre. Jokingly, I phoned him and asked if he'd slept with another woman before I'd flown down there. I wasn't ready for the answer.

''Yes, I did and I felt too guilty to tell you.''

Anger and rage poured into the phone. ''How could you do this to me you . . . . Didn't I tell you any infection would set me way back or end my life? I'm immune compromised.''

Blankly he said, ''You already had fever blisters on your mouth, so I didn't think it would hurt you because you already had them.''

''I didn't have *her* particular strain of virus, you a.....e.''

What can one say to that kind of ignorance? Jean-Pierre was now only a convenience to me to survive the trip back home. Cold rage locked in my body towards him.

The goodbyes were difficult for everyone. Amy broke down crying about how sad she was to leave her friends. I cuddled her. She seemed to be coming down with another bladder infection (later on, I discovered her bladder and kidney symptoms were allergic reactions to ice cream!).

Sherry hugged me and cried with me. Fr. Peter, who helped me to forgive myself and let in the peace, blessed me, then left me in God's hands after a huge hug. Vera, my three-times-a-week employee, who'd been leaving me emotionally a little at a time, grabbed me, hugged me and blurted out, "I'll miss you." I'll miss you too, Vera. She was a rock when I needed it and I her rock, her humor for a marital split-up. Friends. Painful to let go. And I said goodbye to her, that part of me that I would leave behind in Berkeley. My time there was immortalized in the poem, *Berkeley, I never knew you.*

>I entered your portals
>>across the Bay
>the promise of Frisco
>>a bridge away
>But fate was determined
>>to have its way
>Berkeley, I never knew you
>
>Glancing out my glass prison window
>>Seeing the city of my dreams
>>>locked away from me
>By illness too cruel to exist
>
>>The illusion of the theaters,
>parks, the Wharf
>>Only a bridge away
>A deadly bridge away
>
>For toxins englass my body
>>Removing me from life
>>Through glass I look
>>But cannot go in
>
>Berkeley you're famous
>>for radicalism
>>>Stop the canal
>>>>death penalty
>>>>>impeach Reagan
>Walking 'round in tattered clothes
>>Espousing noble aims
>Berkeley, I never knew you
>
>Are the souls real here
>>Are their hearts true
>>Or covered with fuzz
>>Unable to see through?
>
>But Berkeley I hardly know you
>>Yet you know of me
>>>A part I was without entering

The move to Santa Monica was successful. The 45 minute airplane ride went fine. As I was measuring the nystatin out on my kitchen spoon to take a dose, the stewardess came up to me.

"What is that?"

"Nystatin powder."

"What's it for?"

"A systemic fungus infection."

Laughing to myself, I knew she might have thought I'd cleverly disguised cocaine as a yellow powder. When I showed her the prescription label, she relaxed. So curious had she become, she asked me about my disease. I regaled her with my horror story the rest of the flight. Little did she know talking to her helped me make it through the flight without intense terror of what might happen to me. Another blessing.

Jean-Pierre picked us up at Orange County Airport, a tiny one where I didn't have to deal with the amount of diesel fumes at L.A. International. Burying my true feelings toward him, I greeted him cheerily telling him how glad I was he could pick us up.

The move went very smoothly despite the 100° weather and second stage smog alert. The movers had to be all non-smokers, for smoke on peoples' clothing sent me into shock (this happened in Berkeley — we were detained 24 hours while the company found a new crew!).

On the fourth day of my arrival, the fog rolled in. My body started reacting on paint and new wood outdoors. A man smoking on the street 20 feet away gave me chest pain. I became really depressed. Was the move a mistake? Jean-Pierre tried to reassure me but I couldn't be. I wanted to die again for the 90th time that year. Everytime Jean-Pierre came near me, all I could do was cry. For in Santa Monica, Erlander was my only help. No doctors knew the disease in the terminal stage.

I attempted one cup of the taheebo diluted into sips. Once again faintness and dizziness gripped me. Stopped again. Too much for my body right now along with the nystatin.

On September 14, I upped one dose of nystatin to gr 1/16. In the meantime, I continued using garlic, parsley and onion to control the candida. Garlic kills fungus and has natural selenium which builds up the body's defenses. Parsley is a detoxifier, and full of Vitamin C, which I couldn't take; onions also kill fungus.

A new condition presented itself in Santa Monica — the dreaded Santa Ana winds. These are dry, hot winds which blow from inland to the ocean, carrying massive amounts of chemicals and pollens. They are usually accompanied by stagnant air. Normal people feel uncomfortable; the allergic person, whether suffering from classic allergies — trees, weeds etc.

— or chemical, can be severely affected by them. Positive ions, the body destroyer, are in abundance in this condition. The sensitive individual will experience anything from mild irritation to migraines, severe agitation and suicidal depressions. My response was the insane suicidal depressions. Peanuts to the rescue. Head tight, viselike all day. To protect myself I ran my filter and air conditioner continuously along with a negative ionizer and stayed indoors: most of my symptoms were alleviated. Immunplex relieved the fogged brain. Complicating an already bad situation, Malibu, just north of me, was experiencing massive brush fires that turned the air into hydrocarbon heaven. Yet I survived all that. Something was definitely working.

My relationship with Jean-Pierre wasn't. I dumped him again on September 11. I vowed to myself I'd never spend another birthday or holiday with him, for he'd always deserted me to spend them with his nearly ex-wife and little girls. I had enough to deal with, I told myself, I refused to allow any person, place, or thing set me back. This included him. My birthday was enjoyed with my children and their little friends plus my surrogate mother from Ireland, Theresa. Life was looking up.

We celebrated at the Palisades. Cliffs several hundred feet high overlook the serene Pacific Ocean about two miles west of my house. Here, on this strip of grass and trees atop the cliff, dubbed Palisades Park, I replaced the Berkeley Pier for my daily clean air walks. This discovery lessened my sense of isolation for there were many people there, especially young men, walking or jogging for me to talk to. I spent the rest of September and October walking the Palisades and gabbing with men. No one believed how sick I was. One of them unpacked my entire house; another fixed broken closet doors. Flirting was a pleasure, as long as they stayed downwind with the aftershave and shampoo. Some semblance of being in the world, a part of life again, was given to me there. It saved my sanity.

As I was becoming more and more well, my notes were scantier and scantier. Weeks passed without a word written. That always meant good days. Life was definitely better back in Santa Monica, for I didn't feel the dreadful isolation and loneliness as acutely as I had in Berkeley where all my contacts, people-wise, were survival oriented. But I still was severely isolated. Neither my children nor I could have friends in. Shampoo and conditioner still sent me into shock just by my opening the front door to someone who had used them. Unlike Berkeley, I didn't seem to know anybody here who didn't wash his hair.

Toward late September I raised the dose of nystatin again to gr $\frac{1}{16}$. Shoulder pain ensued but was liveable. More green stools and bloating. The bloating with nystatin arrives daily as the drug kills off candida. A lot of gas and foam is formed — just like a beer head. Usually it's passed rectally but can be reabsorbed from the intestines into the bloodstream, causing more flu symptoms. Colonics are helpful, but at this stage, I was unable to tolerate instilling plain water into my intestines, for this left me weak and faint.

September was truly a blessed month. Sweating, that normal everyday bodily function we take for granted, began again. Sweating was something I'd ceased to do for several years. Without it, the body toxins build up to a fatal overload. Again, I was in awe I continued to be alive! I cried with joy at this progression.

I cried with despair when Amy said ''my head itches'' and I discovered head lice in her hair. Jen had them too. The only effective treatment for bugs is a toxic pesticide shampoo. *Good God, no; I'll kill Jean-Pierre.* A week earlier his two little ones had slept over. Their heads were itching then. *I'll kill him.*

''Jean-Pierre the girls have lice.''

''So do mine. My wife just called from Palo Alto to inform me she found them when they got home.''

''You knew they had itchy heads and you brought them here?''

No reply. The only thought in my head besides amputating his was the job in front of me to wash all the bedding to prevent further infestation. That, on top of using someone else's house to wash their hair with the lice shampoo, for the pesticide fumes could be fatal to me.

Jean-Pierre's house was perfect. Not only would I feel better that he assisted in the lices' demise, but he could risk getting them himself instead of me. Selfish you say? Revenge and self-preservation I say. He agreed to the job.

In October, I ate a nectarine. ''Nothing happened.'' My first taste of fruit in over a year. When I could raise the dose of nystatin without the severe side effects previously recorded, I knew I'd make a great deal of progress. That over, a new challenge came along simultaneously — the driver's license renewal.

I'd stalled the DMV long enough with letters for special requests on renewing my license. They turned me down cold. I had to use all my ingenuity to figure out how to take the exam without going into the building. At last, there was a sympathetic supervisor, who hearing I got asthma from perfume and cigarette smoke (a little fudging here — one does have to give ''normies'' a diagnosis they can comprehend) said, ''Bring me a doctor's note and I'll let you take the test outside supervised by an official of the DMV.'' Great! Another obstacle overcome. The doctor was very cooperative with the note, so the date was set for November 5.

We hit another session of Santa Anas. The air pockets in Westwood by UCLA are the most polluted with this condition I discovered, as I went there for one hour, and collapsed, feeling as if I'd smoked marijuana — high as a kite and giggling. Nightmares plagued me all though this period along with the die-off symptoms. Present experience taught me to lower the dosage to the lowest one can when heavily exposed to chemicals. Grains 1/32 four times a day was my maintenance dose.

Huge brush fires cursed Santa Monica again. So many homes burned in Malibu, complete with plastic accoutrements, that the air became like a five-alarm fire over the entire area. I could not go out at all, for dizziness combined with blacking out felled me. Crushing vise-like headaches besieged me for nine days. I'd call Zena in agony threatening to bash my brains out on a wall. All I could do was lie on the floor and cry in pain. Nothing worked against the density of these hydrocarbons — filters, ionizers, immunplex, sealed room. I had to survive — that's all — without committing suicide. Obviously, I did.

Throughout this Jean-Pierre would show up occasionally, blabbing about how tough his life was and dripping in self-pity. His negative personality was draining me more and more every day. *God, I prayed, please strengthen my body so I won't need him anymore.*

After the smoke fumes ended, the exposures, the collapses, the feeling good for several days, the candida die-off went on and on in an endless circle. Tar fumes across the street caused me to collapse in my sealed home. Salvation came at the Palisades, breathing the ocean air when the Santa Anas were absent. My life revolved around this little park for the next two years. It became my life both physically and socially, thereby saving my sanity. Sunshine, fresh air and walks have a tremendous healing effect upon the body along with the other parameters. Throughout October, more and more improvements were added to my list!

ate chinese food — no reaction
tried persimmon — mild craziness
sausage and eggs — no reaction
fixed up house and hung pictures — high energy day
tried bacon — seems okay (fresh)
chopped meat and beans — snitched a little
fever blisters — crazy a little

By October 30, I'd been on three doses of gr 1/16 since the past Sunday. Barely able to function. Sleeping ten-twelve hours a day. (Candida die-off always produces a great need for extra sleep — a very positive sign.)

The air quality had been very good for several days which helped a great deal. November was nearing — the great season of clear air in L.A., for the most part, through April or May. Five months of this would be enormously advantageous in my healing.

I was able to attend an outdoor art fair. My morale was going up, up, up. Of course I had to dodge cigarette smoke and all chemicals as usual but I was participating in life a wee bit and I believe this too helped my healing course.

Again, I dumped Jean-Pierre. The pain of abandonment hit me once more. As sad as I was to be all alone, I was beginning to see how adversely he affected my physical status, which meant my brain was clearing sufficiently to see some truth. When I was dying, I had to block out reality. I paid physically. However, other things balanced me and I healed, despite all this physical stress.

A simple solution helped me to deal with the emotional stress which immediately sent my body into collapse. I asked myself instantly, "Is this person, place or thing worth my health?" *No* was always the immediate answer. This change of attitude would prove beneficial in turning the whole disease around, for letting go of everyday turmoil freed my energy to heal my body. A great lesson.

November came. And moo shu pork. And unscented body oil. No reaction. We'd hit the rainy season. Positive ions are very concentrated before a storm. I could always tell when one was coming — agitation, anger, weepy. As soon as one drop of rain fell, I felt great. For rain releases negative ions, producing the smell of fresh mountain air. Here in California we are now dealing with acid rain at intervals. So the positive ions don't always disseminate, but usually do, leaving me feeling wonderful and full of energy.

Gas poisoning came on November 18 as I was trying to convert my home to all electric. After carefully explaining to a male acquaintance not to allow any gas to escape the gas line when they removed the stove, and not to light a match, he did it anyway. (No one, and I mean no one who does not have this disease, can understand how a person can be so deadly sensitive to anything.)

As I entered the door, he proudly told me how he and the servicemen had checked the line with a match before sealing it. I panicked. How long had they, in their ignorance, left it open? I found out. Dizziness. Severe right-sided chest pain felled me right in front of him. Everything going black. Panicked, I told him my symptoms. "Oh, my mother had chest pain too. You'll be all right." Then he left. Thank God I had a nurse's aide in the house. She was with me but didn't know what to do. I was close to unconsciousness with a blank brain. Collapse, body yellow, fell on bed. Crawled out upstairs patio for air. "Jen, phone him (the male acquaintance). Tell him to call the gas company. Emergency, shut off gas." Jen, only 13, was panic stricken but phoned him. "You call for her," he told this young child. "He won't help mom." Blacking out, I had the aide put an emergency call into the gas company. "Be right out." Half-alive, I stumbled outside and lay on the front seat of my car.

The gas man arrived. "What's wrong?" Yellow, gasping, oxygen running, slurred speech, semi-conscious. "Disconnect the gas, I'm allergic to it."

"No one is allergic to gas."

"They are!" I screamed. "Turn it off!"

"I'm not authorized to go in the house."

"Listen, sir, please, or I'll die. Turn it off outside and check the seal inside." Something must have prompted him to comply. Perhaps my color. He said he'd do it. And he did. (Stig Erlander had been telling me for months to disconnect the two gas fireplaces and the stove, then have them removed, but I didn't listen, so overwhelmed was I by now by my condition, and one more major life-threatening job with no one to help me. He said the lines leaked just enough, though they weren't in use, to affect me adversely. Once again, he was right.)

After the technician left, assuring me there were no gas leaks, I re-entered the house. It seemed better for a while. The gas man had told me the company puts a chemical in the odorless gas to identify the smell. No wonder — a deadly chemical is added to the already deadly gas. The strange part was, I couldn't smell anything — that fooled me. Yet, this also confused me, as his statement was the exact opposite of what I was experiencing. I left my home and drove to the Palisades to recuperate from the gas, gasping for fresh air. For when one can't smell the culprit, one's really at a deficit. Upon returning to the house again a few hours later, I collapsed, becoming confused and insane. By that night, I'd inhaled enough fumes that I was up til 3am with the worst brain toxicity I'd experienced to date. My brain was telling me to get in my car and jump off the cliffs. *Get a machete and decapitate Jean-Pierre.* Terrified of myself, I phoned Zena. "Elizabeth, your voice is strange. You must be in a chemical reaction. I bet there is still gas in that house. Are your windows open?" No. "Open the sliding window. Take an immunplex. Where is your oxygen?" (I had trained her well.) "No," I argued, the muscles around my mouth feeling pulled back by an invisible force til I could barely talk. "Elizabeth listen to me — this is chemical." Somewhere inside me, my true self heard her. Opened the window, took immunplex, tried oxygen. Within twenty minutes, a veil, like a cloud, lifted before my very eyes and I was me again. I began crying.

"Zena, I can't go on like this."

"I know," she said, very sympathetically, "this is a nightmare. But it will pass. There is still gas in that house. Air it out in the morning. Are you all right now?"

"Yes," I said. Thank you. Goodnight. *God bless you Zena.*

November 22, I recorded in my journal:

> "Well, it's over. Another episode of feeling close to death. I'm still here and all right now. Gas poisoning has left me pale and weak, but feeling okay. Tomorrow the electrician comes to install lines for the electric stove. I dread any more intruders coming into my home. What will they bring to kill me, unwittingly? Anxiety is always present for me concerning the house. The need for some repair, the fear it will kill me. Such horrible feelings and alone with them. Jean-Pierre, in my life again, stopped over. Warm and affectionate, but he felt ill himself and went home. Momentarily, I felt abandoned. I feel abandoned if he leaves me to go home and sleep. *God, how abandoned I feel — by You, him and life.* Now, I have to face more strangers to reroute the gas lines in my carport under the house outside for the water. That frightens me after this close call. I'll pray again."

The plumber was uncooperative and uncaring about the care needed to remove the pipes. Absolutely hysterical by now, I went to my knees, begging my Creator for an answer. It came. *Install an electric heater and seal off the lines.* A simple, safe solution.

The electrician was a compassionate soul. Very carefuly, he did the work, then asked me for a date. In my condition, I was flattered and declined graciously, explaining it was impossible, then went to my room and cried over my isolation.

This despair proved a blessing. I felt the time had come to try the Pau D'arco again. Nystatin left me clearer, but isolated and severely vulnerable to heavy chemicals. The time had come for stage II of my healing.

Pau D'arco, Stage 2

December 4, 1982 was D-Day. I stopped nystatin for the day so as not to be overdosed by the combination. Cautiously, I took one ounce of the tea, beginning with a small amount, as I did nystatin. Miracle of miracles — all I felt was mild dizziness and slight faintness along with a tremendous surge of energy. The change was instantaneous. I was able to go Christmas shopping with my girls — Gemco, Toys R Us, and Bullocks. Building interiors smelled normal again, not like petrochemicals. Amy remarked in Gemco, ''Mom, a man is standing next to you with a cigarette and nothing happened to you.'' Seems it was my children who noticed the changes first. We shopped for four hours — an impossible task before the one shot of taheebo!

The first day, I tried four - one ounce shots of taheebo (the irony didn't escape me that shots of alcohol had been replaced by shots of taheebo),with only a slight side effect after the third dose: faintness.

The third day I was able to purchase new cotton sheets with pink and lavender flowers and sleep on them. My chest was clamping that night, but Jen had used scented, regular shampoo and perfumed soap — all scents I was unable to tolerate two days earlier. Not sure what I was reacting to, I checked in with Eve. ''Don't stop the nystatin,'' she said. ''not now. You won't be able to tell if you're going through withdrawal or the dosage of taheebo is too much for you.'' Grateful for her guidance, I resumed nystatin at four doses (gr $\frac{1}{16}$), and dropped taheebo to three ounces. Since this was all experimental, no one knew how much or how little each individual could tolerate. I was the third person to try this experiment. To me, I had nothing to lose. Try this or eventually commit suicide from the isolation. Nystatin, I realized, would only slowly kill candida but not heal the immune system. I believed my prayers were answered. Taheebo seemed the answer.

So impressed was I with the taheebo, I decided to give Amy a small dose. She'd become increasingly allergic to antibiotics from multiple ear infections. (Incidentally, every time I thought I was getting well, *I* dumped Jean-Pierre. He became the barometer for quantum leaps in my recovery. Let him go — now.)

Amy fell to the floor on one jigger. "Mom, I'm going to faint." Her response showed me toxicity had begun in her system. By trial and error, we found one teaspoon a day was her dose. We were going to go through this one together.

Depressions set in the first two weeks on Pau. I finally realized they were the result of killing off the toxins. They came and went like a yo-yo. I would feel sad and cry while simultaneously being exhausted. My legs became leaden and pounded.

Many symptoms occurred those first two weeks. However, they were milder with taheebo — transient and different — than nystatin. For instance, there was aching over the kidney area one day. So I cut down to one ounce temporarily. When heavy fog rolled in, I felt crazy a short time only. Eve even suggested rinsing our hair with it to kill dandruff. By now, I was game for anything. My older daughter suffered from crusting on her scalp which I'd always believed was allergic in origin. She used the taheebo and most of the scaling and dandruff disappeared in one treatment. My hair shone and had some life to it when I rinsed it in the tea. There was not a single commercially available conditioner I could use. Now I had a natural one. Improving my appearance really improved my outlook.

Bloating, gas, and green stools again. Yet the biggest difference with taheebo was the sensation of warmth transiently flowing through different organs of my body: the liver, then the spleen, the pancreas and the adrenals. Eve and I concurred the taheebo worked by detoxifying the blocked organs, thereby allowing the body's own energy to enter that spot and begin bringing it back to life.

New sheets produced intense itching. After washing them two more times in Erlander's washing soda, I could finally use them.

The sleeping was up to 10-12 hours daily. A significant amount of detoxifying. Up and down I went on the dose trying to determine what amount my body could tolerate. Taking the taheebo was an act of faith. Finding the right dosage took wisdom based on experience. That knowledge I earned day by day.

On the eighth day, total exhaustion slipped in. Still, I wouldn't stop taking the tea. I knew it was working due to my boundless energy but I didn't know how much the amount I was taking would affect me. Taheebo works on a cumulative effect — that's why it's necessary to go slowly. Around the second week or even sooner, one knows what dose is correct — except for zanies like me who keep pushing too fast.

I'd been sitting outside the door with my carbon mask at AA meetings (which inside tend to look like smoke-filled barrooms), just to have human contact. Being able to be that close to people and cigarette smoke was a small miracle. I know I overexposed myself to life too fast at this period, but the booster it gave my morale was worth it. In any event, I wouldn't recommend what I did — pushing too far, too fast can encourage a relapse which is characterized by severe exhaustion.

The eighth day, the girls and I also trimmed our Christmas tree. Joyous. Amy was so happy to see me pitching in and playing Christmas Carols that she remarked. "Mom, I've never seen you like this — you're like a kid." *No, Amy, that's right, I've had serial severe illnesses since the fourth year of your life.* She was only 10, yet six years of her young life she'd barely had a parent. We had much to rejoice over. So we went to Sav-On and bought scads of decorations plus miniature pencil sharpeners — all metal — shaped as pianos, cars, slot machines, and workable. A marvelous gift idea for her little friends. We went crazy and bought a whole bunch. Such fun! I couldn't shop at all eight days ago! What a miraculous blessing for me! That day too, Amy met her new violin teacher, an elderly man with a twinkle in his heart and joy in his eyes. We loved him as soon as we saw him.

And I cried every now and then over the demise of my love affair with Jean-.Pierre It's very difficult to let go of an intimate relationship when you are so ill — even if it is deadwood. But the girls hugged and hugged me that night. Amy told me to talk about how I felt, like I'd taught them, and I'd feel better. *How I loved her at that moment!* Love surrounded me. Which helped me to cry and let go of all the miserable Christmases since my divorce and the illness's onset. Tears of joy followed over how much we had to be grateful for that day — my first happy Christmas in many a year.

Meanwhile the leg pounding got worse and worse til I couldn't stand the pain nor sleep. I phoned Eve. She said she'd been through this — exhaustion and leg pain are part of the healing. "Continue Elizabeth. Don't quit. You're doing very well."

By Sunday, the ninth day, I realized I'd been through a minor healing crisis. On Monday, my entire body felt bruised, as if I'd been kicked from end to end. Depression, crying and exhaustion were over. Woozy at AA meeting. Reacting on smoke and perfume. Appetite almost non-existent. More exhaustion. Energy returned at 11pm, plus a rampant sex drive. Maddening.

Three ounces seemed my limit. I called Roz S., the other experimenter. "Keep on, don't quit." Told her all my symptoms were returning — chest tightness, face red, numbness in my hands, itching. "That's good," she said. "It's a healing crisis." *I thought that was over. Wait a minute, that's right — I'm about due.* Crises appear about every two months. I decided to hang in there.

December 14, 1982 — eleven days on Pau — I wrote:

"Going through some very rough water on this tea. Late afternoon, I became violently nauseated, vomiting my dinner. Don't know if it was the fish or the tea. Never really know. I feel awful so I took adrenoplex and minerals. I'm so in the dark about this substance. What's in it?

Meanwhile, common sense tells me to go slowly — especially since it's unknown. What keeps me going *is* the fact that I can go into malls and shops and live a little. So I'll press on. It's now 11 days since I've started the tea and the strength it's given me is remarkable. I've also developed a maddening sex drive and don't have a partner. Isn't that a laugh? I finally have a sex drive and no one to play with! How cruel life seems at times. Of course, I will survive and I am grateful it has returned. I trust the rest will come when it's due.''

That very same day I drove to an outdoor meditation center on Sunset Boulevard that was so moldy, had it been the previous year, I would have collapsed. I didn't. I also visited an old woman friend in her figure-control salon, the one I'd had anaphylaxis in. Mona hugged me warmly, shocked at my hair being so white. ''The disease did this.'' I felt so confused and anxious seeing someone I knew that I blurted out all kinds of sad feelings without realizing how sad I really was. Seeing a ''normal'' person made me more acutely experience my isolation from life. Back home, I fell apart, couldn't talk, feelig only tears pouring from me. Then it passed. *This will improve.* Tears of relief flowed from my heart whenever I could go out, see anyone, or go into a building without collapsing. Each tiny step meant progress.

On December 17, I noted orange coating at the base of my teeth while on the larger doses of Pau D'arco. Amy had orange globules in her stool. I didn't know what it meant. (A year later, Orie Bachechi, inventor of the Kiva process, told me his chemists said it was old penicillin being released from the body.) Both of us had been on a great deal of this drug at different intervals in our life.

Headache, nausea and depression continued. Dose still unclear. Stuffing on peanuts again. So down I almost called Jean-Pierre. In the meantime I worked on building up a support system by phone so I'd feel less alone and cut off from people.

Experienced lots of trapped energy in my body. Pacing. Lustful. Unable to release it. Immunplex calmed down this hyperactivity of my immune system. These symptoms were how I determined over-dosage. So I reduced the amount of Pau to two ounces.

Tried Jean-Pierre one more time. So lonely I called him just to be touched physically. We attempted making love — all I could do was cry. Sex didn't work anymore.

The rampant sex drive continued. Desperate, I sat outside the door of an AA meeting again. It helped tremendously.

Normal stools appeared on December 20th. Three ounces was now my maintenance dose plus the nystatin (gr $\frac{1}{16}$ four times a day). I tried chinese food again — body bloated but no cerebrals. Progress.

Jean-Pierre appeared out of nowhere at midnight on December 23rd to tell me he was leaving for Paris for the holidays.

''I wanted to give you your Christmas presents,'' he said softly. Since I'd found out last month he'd been giving his almost ex-wife Christmas and birthday presents behind my back throughout our relationship, I'd made up my mind never to share a holiday or present with him again. *I was through.* As lonely as Christmas might be without him, it would be lonelier to be with him. There was nothing there for me now but hatred and rage toward him.

Jean-Pierre handed me a book written by a psychiatrist, *Fathers and Daughters.* The theme was the importance of having a loving father in a girl's life. Jean-Pierre knew mine had been a brutal relationship. The book struck like a knife. I threw it at him. This didn't stop him. He handed me a blank tape. ''I bought a record for you but I didn't have time to tape it because I had to buy presents for my nieces and nephews.'' The tape *was* our relationship. ''Get out.'' He wanted my blessing. I refused to speak to him. At 3am, he left dejectedly for his 5am plane. Good riddance to bad rubbish I said to myself as I burst into tears.

Christmas Eve was a brighter day. The girls and I shopped for last-minute Christmas gifts. Amy and I stopped in St. Martin of Tours Church to see the manger. I was able to stay despite the lit candles. Another blessing.

Christmas Day proved to be the best one of my entire life for I wrote joyously in my diary:

> ''Today possessed so many major changes in my life that I'm exhausted! I was functioning physically, mentally and spiritually for the first time in six years; I was able to take my girls for a walk and prepare them a bacon and egg breakfast. We fed the birds leftover rye and wheat bread as their Christmas breakfast; I drove my girls through Pacific Palisades. Amy wanted to buy a house because she saw the real estate signs, exclaiming, 'They're on sale!'
>
> Woodsmoke was very heavy throughout the air that day. We ventured to our favorite Chinese restaurant where we enjoyed seven different dishes of which we ate only half; of which I continued to demolish after the girls left [that night] for their vacation with their dad. My first trip to a restaurant in 15 months! That alone would be enough to celebrate. I actually ate *in* the restaurant. My face turned red and I felt a bit faint at times, breaking into a cold sweat, but I did it — that's all that mattered.''

Later on that day, we dropped in to see Theresa, the girls' adopted Eire-born grandmother. This was the second time in two days I'd been in a gas heated house. Strong perfume and her husband's old cigarette smoke had little reaction at all on me.

I know this is anticlimactic but, not once did I mention I was lonely that day, nor utter Jean-Pierre's name. For I had vowed to myself as an act of love that this would be a wonderful Christmas without him. It was.

My worst problem was craving for a cigarette at 9pm and bloating myself with cups of comfrey tea — that was it. This day brought a great deal of healing to me and my family.

The week alone swept swiftly by. Energy was my middle name. Well enough to write. Wanting to be a writer, I ran off a quick article on E.I. for a women's magazine. Tears stained the words. *But I did it.* I tried running for 5 minutes. Although quickly winded, *I did it*. Nausea, fever blisters and bruised feeling all over my body. More candida die-off. I'd upped the dose to four jiggers. Too much. Down to three. Lowered nystatin to gr $\frac{1}{32}$ AM dose. Felt like experimenting. What if I lower nystatin and increase the taheebo? I desperately wanted to get off nystatin because I didn't like the side effects. Passed more mucous and green stools. *That's always a good sign.* Sensations of heat passed through my upper legs, left side, and upper arms at night; Eve had experienced these too: we both felt it was energy entering our devitalized organs.

Friday evening, I was in so much emotional pain, I was back at the altar at St. Martin's asking the Lord to heal me. Many tears fell in that church that night. I felt better. An AA meeting would help. I stood outside a smoke-filled room hoping to see a familiar face. Pat L saw me. We hugged and shared our lives. A fellow AA, named Jim said ''You shouldn't be alone tonight.'' I didn't know what he meant. Later on, we sat in my den gabbing. If Amy hadn't called at midnight to see if I were dead, I'd never have known it was New Year's Eve. Can you believe it — *I thought it was the next day!* I wished the girls a happy New Year, yelling and screaming into the phone joyfully with them. Jean-Pierre called from Paris. I allowed my answering machine to take the call. I realized I would be all right alone; Jim was the one who needed me. Kindly, I sent him home. A new year had begun.

Nineteen eighty three brought rapid progress on the Pau D'arco. The list of things I could use and eat again in January was lengthy: ice cream, face moisturizer, makeup, lipstick, body oil, wash clothes in Borax, eggs, sausage at a restaurant. The physical changes were more dramatic! Chest only tightening from smoke, no viselike pain, and going to many affairs — all previously impossible for me!

Simultaneously, the physical healing symptoms became more interesting. A maddening itch persisted for three nights (felt it was toxins coming through the skin). More fever blisters and pustules in my mouth. (I believe this is a result of candida die-off). Small hives and rash on abdomen — transient. Severe hunger disappeared when I discontinued my B vitamins. Thank God — for I'd put on 15 pounds in two weeks — a great change from an inability to gain weight. Now I was fat! Seemed my body had begun producing its own nutritional needs when nystatin worked. Abdominal bloating and green stools. Perspiring during love making (Jean-Pierre was in my life again for a while). Perspiration is a true sign the body can begin detoxifying itself, and a very significant indication that the disease is turning around. Whoopee!

The end of January brought a huge healing crisis. And torrential rains which caused my carport to be flooded four times in one week with one to three feet of water. Mold grew freely in this atmosphere. I collapsed. Half-conscious, I hired a young fellow to scrub the walls down with Borax. It helped. The combination, I'm sure, protracted the healing crisis. It went on for a record three weeks.

The desire to heal rapidly reached its peak in January. So desperate was I to be through with all this, for the toll it was taking on my children, that I decided to try something new — a psychic healer.

The healer I met had been through a near-death experience whereby he "came back" having the gift of healing. Still, I was very skeptical of him, thinking this a little bit of witchcraft and a bunch of malarkey.

But I tried it anyway. After the "healing", whereby I felt heat from his hands on my abdomen and cold in the kidney - adrenal area, I became very weak. The next day I felt limp around cigarette smoke. My left arm became numb and colorless, likewise the left leg, followed by generalized weakness. The healer said "weakness follows a healing." Exhausted. Washed my hair — red spotting on my face, shoulders and forearms. Scared. Added extra dose of Pau D'arco. Large green stool. Weakness in left arm. Mild left shoulder pain. I had three massages that week. Massage helps loosen and pull toxins out of the tissues and increase circulation to the lymphatics. It also feels good. It's being touched.

All my old symptoms were returning. This happens in a healing crisis as you kill off the toxins. Up and down I went. This episode began on January 24. On February 1, when I had a good day, I became overconfident and ate, of all things, a piece of frozen pizza. This was right after I'd gone to check my moldy basement from the flood, from which I developed a horrible depression with crying, on and off, all day.

Severe chemical reactions began that day: depression, crying, apathy, numbness in my left arm, violent rage, color waxen, and blue nails in my left hand. Felt as if I were dying around 4pm. Prayed and prayed for God's strength. I fell asleep. Then came slurred speech. Acute alcoholic intoxication symptoms. "Not fair, Lord," I cried out in anguish, "I haven't had a drop."

The pizza engendered the worst healing crises of my entire recovery. Highlights are presented here so you will know what to expect and also benefit by my mistakes:

> *February 1, 1983:* Legs pounding . . . severe weakness, became violent, punching walls, locked self in bedroom so as not to harm children . . . called therapist for help . . . Crying uncontrollably, called Roz S. in Hayward. "Cheese acted like antibiotics, Elizabeth" . . . Made sense . . . Wasted . . . miserable.
>
> 2/2/83   Color poor . . . Intestines burning . . . Weak. Massage — helped . . . Saw Jean-Pierre . . . Orgasm brought on entire body turning red and burning . . . then shaking chills (wonder

how I could make love when I'm dying — you really enjoy the moment!) Can't stand up . . . Pain left shoulder. 12 pm - passed large green stool . . . Color improved. Felt much better . . Talked to Eve . . . ''Cheese is bad news,'' (no kidding) . . . Air clean . . . Felt stronger.

2/4 Faint. Collapsing . . . Food cravings maddening . . . . Stuffing on food and peanuts. Large brown stool this AM. Weak. Inability to think. Felt like I had a general anesthetic . . . Slept 11 hours.

2/5 Rained all day . . . Felt I was taking too much medicine. Cut Pau D'arco completely . . . Insane sex drive (hypothalmus overstimulation). Cut nystatin to 3 doses gr 1/16. Stuffed on chicken livers and peanuts. Vomited. Headache, sad, depressed.

2/8 Rough, rough days. Crying, depression, severe weakness, mind foggy, unable to maintain train of thought. Called doctor. Blood drawn for electrolytes and blood chemistries. Petechiae (broken blood vessels) on right upper inner surface of arm. Reacting to gas heat (in stores). Chest Pain. Collapsed in doctor's office. Crawled home . . . . Doctor phoned, ''Take potassium gluconate.'' Got some. Nauseated, vomited. Felt worse after each dose of tea and nystatin. Confused . . . Usually feel better after medicine . . . Haven't recovered from cheese, flooding and psychic healing . . . Short walks helped . . . Too weak to move much. Some moter aphasia (loss of speech) . . . Loss of comprehension. Inability to complete sentence. Short term memory loss. Waxen color, coldness left arm alternating to right arm then disappearing (old, old symptoms.) Phoned doctor . . . 'Take four potassium pills' . . . Severe nausea and fainting.

2/9 Sickness appears over . . . Slept 9½ hours. Awoke feeling O.K. . . . Blood test normal. Amazing . . . Massage . . . Severe tenderness left shoulder, arm and big toe. Tried potassium again — nausea and headache. Started minerals again.

The healing crisis ended February 12. Nineteen days. Believe me, I reached despair during this one. Without Zena and Jean-Pierre's support, I wouldn't have made it. This event was the second worst I'd experienced in my journey. It took a lot out of me but I learned a lot of lessons which I'll share with you in order that you may be spared what I went through.

First, I don't know what the influence was of the psychic healing but would be more cautious about it if I chose to do it again.

Second, Pau D'arco must be stopped during a crisis and the nystatin kept at a minimum maintenance dose to control the candida growth. One goes back to the original dose they could tolerate in the initial taking of nystatin.

Third — don't push to go up on the dose too rapidly. The result can be serious.

And last of all, I learned I cannot heal any faster than I am healing. Patience. This one was trying my soul.

My healing crisis, I want to reassure you, is not the usual — it was extreme. However, the longer you've been sick or the more seriously ill you are, the slower you must go. This is fact. you did not become ill overnight; you will not heal overnight.

The good news after a healing crisis is you feel great and are able to do more. Why, even my relationship with Jean-Pierre underwent a change. I decided to keep Jean-Pierre as a friend who could help me when the chips were down — that's all. Otherwise, we were totally incompatible. He was always loving and supportive emotionally at these times. I couldn't forget this. Once again, I decided to overlook his glaring faults and confusion. Some clarity was entering my life.

Now I was able to stay in a meeting room of approximately 100 people! No longer did I black out from perfume and aftershave. Only a little dizziness, some anger and redness of my face. The crisis healed me deeply; it also made me fat, for the food cravings drove me to eat and eat. *Twenty pounds*. Depressing. But a small price to pay for being alive. I would have to remind myself of that fact, time and time again, throughout the next year.

Another conference with Eve on February 16th. Seemed my symptoms were returning. She said, ''Try going up to gr ⅛.'' Eve also reminded me to try bee pollen again. ''Bee pollen provides the essential amino acids which are necessary to the body's functioning at all. I used it because I couldn't tolerate any commercial brand — all petrochemical.'' (At a later date, I did try unsprayed bee pollen — no difference for me — but could help others in earlier phases to reduce chemical reactions.) Just juggling the nystatin dose was enough for me at that time.

Within three days on gr ⅛, I was symptom free again. By Sunday I had chest pain and pressure in my lungs when I was exposed to cigarette smoke. Monday I increased the 2pm dose to gr ⅛. The reactions were diminishing. Tuesday I added more to the 11am dose. I felt better and better. The reactions were almost absent Wednesday. I changed the morning dose to gr ⅛. Day was excellent. Normal energy. I was also taking three ounces of Pau D'arco. The food cravings disappeared. At this juncture I felt I'd reached another major turning point. For I shopped briefly in a supermarket without any reactions. The air was extremely moldy and humid. I felt fine.

In fact, so well, I attended a HEAL* meeting where I announced the miracle of taheebo as a possible answer to our dilemma. Sufferers were very grateful and listened. The president of the chapter invited me to a HUXLEY meeting the following week, a group for people diagnosed as psychiatric who actually had chemical or food allergies.

*HEAL - Human Ecology Action League

Ann Melton, a young physician, was the speaker. Her talk was inspiring. Not only did she have the affliction herself but she had a comprehension of the physical and mental ramifications. This was a major breakthrough in my isolation to find a physician who comprehended my plight. This fact alone alleviated my intense feeling of isolation. For although, I could go ''out'' more and more, I was still very limited to where I could go ''in'' (buildings, that is). Coming into my home at all remained nearly impossible for shampoo and conditioner were still my major enemies.

Excited beyond belief, I raised my hand to tell Ann I was a ''universal reactor'' with pan anaphylaxis. She blanched. ''You have great courage,'' she said, ''to even be here.'' ''Yes, thank you, Dr. Melton. I also have Pau D'arco which I believe heals the immune system.'' She'd not heard of it. I told her I'd fill her in after the meeting, which I did. A friend. I'd made a friend. Ann invited me to a talk she was giving the following evening to the clinical ecologists. Delightedly I accepted, despite the fact that the thought of going into an unknown restaurant terrified me.

On February 23, I went to Ryan's to hear Dr. Melton address other physicians on our disease. (I used a carbon mask to survive the candles on the tables and used oxygen to clear out my head when I arrived home.) She was dynamite. Many of the doctors found it hard to believe anything so horrifying could exist. I verified her observations. And was bombarded afterward by two doctors asking me questions. This liaison gave me a real shot in the arm. Meeting Ann gave me a connection on my level of knowledge. Grateful, I looked forward to more contact.

By February 28 my body had adjusted to the higher doses of nystatin. The severe peanut cravings and weight gain began again. Now I was full of energy and didn't know what to do with it. So I saw Jean-Pierre that night. It was O.K. Nothing special. His occasional visits were just O.K. I hoped someone with a full deck would enter my life soon.

Tornadoes, earthquakes, and torrential rains struck southern California the week of March 1. Garage flooded again. Head was tightening. Nausea. However, generally speaking, full of boundless energy. Seemed a lot had changed since last month. Adding small amounts of taheebo alleviated the food cravings. And the weight gain kept on.

Lumped together with these problems was acute Jean-Pierre withdrawal, for I saw less and less of him trying to wean myself of him and let go, for both our sakes. That night I fell to the floor pounding out my rage at God for my terrible plight, but especially for the lack of human contact. *I hated Him.* Without two friends — Zena to listen to my pain and Jean-Pierre to hold me — I don't know if I'd have had the will to survive. You can't make it through this ailment alone!

Tuesday, March 8, I got a bright idea! Why not go off nystatin and take Pau D'arco solo? Then, I reasoned, I'll have that added chemical out of my body and I'll heal faster. Great thought, wrong approach.

Two days off nystatin, while continuing on six ounces of taheebo, I was besieged with headaches, depression, and increasingly severe left shoulder pain. Three days off nystatin, the shoulder pain subsided. Anxiety and fear plagued me. Desire to crawl under covers, not think. The slightest pressure too much. Weird ups and downs. Taking a few doses here and there. Eve warned me, ''I wouldn't just cut nystatin Elizabeth.'' The doctors knew less than we about withdrawal, so I was on my own. Scary. Challenging. Weakness, faintness, nausea, and headaches ensued. By Monday, I was severely agitated. So I went to the Palisades for my walk where a ''voice'' told me to jump off; ''life was useless.'' Oh, no — *that voice.* Despair is a toxic reaction to mold. Holding my head, I flew in my car back home. Shaken, I called Dr. Melton. ''You O.D.'d on nystatin. Quit for today.''

Quit for today? That caused a yo-yoing emotionally. I didn't know what to do. Confused and frightened, I went to a huge AA meeting and stood outside. I felt like a newcomer (a newly sober alcoholic) with all the symptoms of withdrawal. The problem was — I hadn't been drinking. AA had taught me any drug after one becomes addicted physically will put one through withdrawal symptoms. This thought comforted me. Surprisingly, I noted I was in smoke and aftershave. *Nothing happened to me.*

Pain began later in the left side of the back of my head. Sex drive hyper, and agitation again. In between all this, I'd worked with Zena with whom I consulted in her backyard (only place I could survive in her terrain), releasing deep pain of abuse by my father during childhood illnesses. Needless to say, I was under severe stress.

And so it went through that week. On and off nystatin. Up and down on Pau D'arco. A horrible brain reaction started at midnight that Sunday — terror, paranoia, crying, afraid of everything. Felt myself fading. Dying feeling again. At 11pm, I took a dose of nystatin, gr $\frac{1}{32}$, then passed a green stool right after ingesting the drug. The symptoms were alleviated.

The very next day total confusion set in — I could not remember if I did or didn't take nystatin. Didn't know what to do. Low clouds, high humidity (86°). Miserable day. Perfect for candida growth; perfect for memory loss.

March 18, I wrote in my journal:

> ''Cutting nystatin is a no-no as the withdrawal is worse than anything I have experienced, including coming off alcohol. Monday evening, I had sheer terror and diarrhea. Zena was my lifeline. Tuesday, I had shaking chills, nausea and headaches. Then the symptom to end all symptoms — the muscles of my jaw, face, and neck became tauter and tauter, as if someone had a hook behind my head and was pulling the muscles and nerves out through the back of my head while twisting the hook to tighten it more and more. Before I ran through the glass window and jumped off the second-floor patio, I phoned Dr. Melton. It was 12 midnight.

Ann told me to stay off nystatin. And, I belonged in an ecology unit. Ignoring her advice, I took an immunplex and came out of it.

After I hung up, it began again. So I took a small dose of nystatin, gr $\frac{1}{32}$ — immediately relaxed, and fell asleep.

That was the answer. I relate this in great detail, again not to scare you, but to inform you that these symptoms are withdrawal and can be alleviated by a small dose. I warn you strongly from my experience *never* to cut nystatin. Again, my symptoms were extreme, due to the complication of genetically severe alcohol and drug sensitivities, but I do know of others who've suffered this way. So I pray my knowledge will prevent others from going through so frightening an experience.

Dr. Melton was so concerned about me mentally, that she advised me to put in an emergency call to a psychologist, a Dr. Bain, who had the disease and with whom she worked out of Escondido. She needed to assess my emotional state professionally to best assist me in my course. I told her I had a therapist whom I trusted, but agreed to see Dr. Bain if he could come to my home.

Bain was speaking in Brentwood that night. He'd meet me afterwards. I attended his talk. He really knew the toxic brain symptoms cold. When he arrived at my home, he was amazed I could wear lipstick. "Got that back in December," I told him. He asked me to describe the illness at its worst. "Pananaphylaxis" I said, "for three weeks." He dropped his pencil "May I ask you a question? — I don't know how you're alive! How did you do it?" "God," I said quietly.

When he recovered from his shock, Bain told me a person reaching my state took eight *years* for the immune system to turn around, if they stayed alive, that is. Mine had done it in a year and a half. He was speechless. He asked me to tell him again how I did it. I laughed then briefly mentioned prayer and Pau D'arco. He left a transformed man.

Thursday, St. Patrick's Day, bravely, I drove an hour southbound to get my girls haircut by our old beautician. Upon reaching Redondo Beach I realized I always felt depressed as I hit this area where I formerly lived. Why it was *the refineries* on either side of my home in Palos Verdes that had caused the depressions! *My reaction was chemical!* What a revelation! It freed me of chronic depressed feelings about the area. A black cloud descended upon me whenever I went there. So that was the explanation — petrochemical poisoning. This fact freed me of thinking my depressions were emotional when I lived in Palos Verdes. They were too pervasive to be real.

The return drive went without incident. After an extremely traumatic week, I decided to spend a weekend healing myself, doing merry things for me. I'd had too much surviving and too little love. It's called "filling up." And so I did, until Sunday night which rejuvenated me and gave me the strength to deal with what was in front of me. For Sunday night, like a pumpkin, I became a Mom again when the girls returned from their Dad's. Boy, did I need energy for that!

The next few weeks I spent in deep mourning for the past tragedies in my life that led up to making me so sick. A lack of love as a child, including deep rage and anger at the abuse I'd suffered, had eventually culminated in so serious a malady. A healing crisis, physical though it is, releases deeply depressed rage, which otherwise wouldn't come to the surface. As horrible as the physical reactions are, they can work for you in your healing!

Again, I tried to go off nystatin: grain $\frac{1}{32}$ during the day, gr $\frac{1}{16}$ at night, two jiggers of Pau D'arco. Still too much for my body. At the same time, Dr. Erlander informed me he'd devised a new washing product combining his washing soda with pure baking soda. When I washed my clothing with the new compound, they were less gray and had no reaction on my skin. Another advance!

Once more, I believed, I was well enough to go off nystatin; what I didn't know is that withdrawal produces heightened chemical sensitivity for a short period of time. Full of confidence, I walked into a store to buy vacuum cleaner bags. The man was using cleaning fluid. Difficulty breathing, severe headache ... nausea ... dizziness. Fell out of store ... drove home ... oxygen for 15 minutes ... two immunplex ... craved carbohydrates ... ate ice cream ... depression ... crying jag.

That Saturday, March 26, I awakened with swollen eyes and gray eyeballs — symptoms of acute toxicity of the kidneys. That same afternoon, two men delivered a book case I had had made from formaldehyde-free wood. One had on aftershave. As I was collapsing to the floor, the other remarked comically, "This is the crazy lady who thinks she is allergic to everything." Still conscious, I raved at him, "I'm not crazy, I'm sick." I fell past them, dragging myself up to my bedroom on the second floor. Weak ... crying... shocky ... bed with five covers ... and oxygen ... chills ... two immunplex ... fell asleep. Very frightened. At the same time, I discovered a neighbor was using heavy duty cleaning chemicals in our common driveway. *The fumes were all over our house.* The girls closed the windows and turned on all the filters. I fled, in a semi-daze to Jean-Pierre's house, where I was safe. He tucked me in. For the 90th time, I thought *this is it, I'm going to die.* All I could do was cry.

A journal entry on April 2, sums up this exposure:

"I'm still here. Survived chemical exposures. Came out of it in three days. Stabilized on nystatin past week — four doses gr $\frac{1}{16}$ plus three ounces Pau D'arco. Santa Ana condition yesterday. Only slight nausea and headache. Tightness in shoulders and neck all day."

To recover from a severe poisoning in three days was great progress. Previously, the course had been two weeks or more. These continuing improvements, despite the suffering, gave me the courage to go on. The good days were becoming more and more, the bad days less and less. A light was beginning to shine at the end of the tunnel.

Eve came up with some more news on how to detoxify. She'd heard of a procedure whereby you used baking soda baths. Knowing Eve can overdo anything and I can't, I tried the baking soda — half the amount. The water turned murky. Toxins were pulled out of me. However, I began itching from the baking soda. Great improvement from when it placed me in shock. I never tried the rest — the baking soda was potent enough.

Easter came and went. Did I forget to mention I dumped Jean-Pierre again? (for the 50th time). By now this affair had become humorous. It would make a great movie! The only way I could be with him was to join him in his let's pretend phoniness. With clarity entering my life more and more, and healing progressing, I could see him more clearly. Wasn't nice.

On this occasion, he had the audacity to ask me to stay at his house for a few hours a day, taking phone calls from would-be renters. The rage inside me was so deep I could have called him all sorts of names. I was to do this, while he spent Easter weekend with his almost ex-wife, and kids and her family in Palm Springs!

To add insult to insult, he let himself into my house and left flowers — tulips — on my bed, with an innocuous note — "Love Jean-Pierre" — and an ad for his rental! *Such nerve.* My first plan was to throw the flowers through the front window of his house. My second, I did! I delivered them back to his house, throwing the pot at the light beige, carpeted stairs with a note of goodbye and good riddance (again). Seeing the splattered dirt on the new carpeting avenged my heart. To have this stress on top of being so ill was too horrible for words. Yet, I still had anaphylaxis. Until that no longer existed, I would need him to drive my limp body from my chemically toxic house during an exposure. *And he knew it too. I was a victim. That was my reality.*

As I got well, overlooking Jean-Pierre's madness became more and more difficult. I prayed to God to help me. The answer came in an unusual way — not right away; I'll get into that at a later date. Meanwhile writing became a major outlet for my frustration.

Writing out one's advances in recovery lifts the spirits.

On April 8, 1983 I wrote:

Changes physically in past week:

1) night urination stopped (I forgot to mention one voids small amounts all night in acute phase)
2) abdomen not swelling unless I eat peanuts or sprouted beans.

3) peanut cravings almost ceased
4) only when exposed to large amount of hydrocarbons —
   smoke-filled rooms — crave peanuts
5) able to tolerate ascorbic acid (Vitamin C) — no fever blisters
   or inflammation of gums.
   (possible small reaction — tightness in neck)

I continued on nystatin, gr $\frac{1}{16}$, plus three ounces taheebo. Intuitively, I knew I'd be off nystatin soon. Since I still had some trouble with Vitamin C, I called Steve Levine for his opinion. He said in the absence of the liver enzyme, glutathione, Vitamin C breaks down into poison. Makes sense. He was in the process of preparing a pure glutathione for people like myself. When available, possibly a few weeks, he'd send me some. I relinquished Vitamin C for now.

I phoned Eve about my progress. She told me she'd found a book named "Survival Factors in the Neoplastic and Viral Diseases" by Dr. William Koch. He was ahead of his time and was persecuted for his work, eventually fleeing the U.S.

"UCLA's Health Science Department had it." she added. Why, UCLA was five minutes from my house. I purchased this highly technical book and read it. Koch had worked with the quinones (one of them, Pau D'arco) successfully, even mentioning treating cases of environmental illness back in the 30's! Amazing. The quinones resurrect the damaged cell, permitting it to regenerate itself through proper oxygenation, was Koch's theory in a nutshell. Intuitively, I knew he was right.

Eve and I discussed this book excitedly, for here was the key to healing E.I. But Koch's procedures were illegal in the U.S. We also consulted with one another on the cause of the bruised body feeling from the taheebo. Eve felt it was salt imbalance or electrolytes which kept the body in synch. Kelp and alfalfa tablets rectified this situation — one per hour till it went away. Alfalfa, combined with 6-8 glasses of water, also helped the dehydration headaches one experiences on Pau D'arco. The headaches, likewise, are caused by too rapid de-tox. Either way, alfalfa or kelp tablets and water relieve these symptoms.

I was so busy learning how to get well, I didn't notice something happening very imperceptibly: I'd become more interested in living than chronicling the illness. I was out of isolation!

For April 28, 1983, my diary states:

My journal's entries are becoming farther and farther apart. Tonight as I suffer some strange pain in my left upper quadrant around the pancreas, I reflect on recent events. Jean-Pierre and I saw "Night of the Shooting Stars," a very moving Italian film about Italy's involvement with Mussolini and Naziism in World War II, and the confusion with each other as to who was on whose side. We played for awhile, then I went home. Seeing him occasionally is the best I can do now, for I am re-entering life, and need someone with me who knows what I've been through as I attempt life once more ....

Earlier that day, I thought I'd have a nervous breakdown, for I'd been unable to hire help for seven or eight weeks. Most of the female aides thought I was crazy or looked at me as if I were possessed, never to return. A friend came to help for one day, a young healthy 25-year-old woman, and was overwhelmed by the restrictions within an hour, then left permanently.

Magic also occurred that day, for I listed *nothing happened* with the below:

Wore old cranberry clothes (some synthetic) — no reaction
Movie with Jean-Pierre — no reaction
Bathed with perfumed soap — no reaction
Made love on Jean-Pierre's bed — no depression
Went to Jen's high school orientation over 500 people — no reaction.

Life was being returned to me.

RE-ENTRY

May 2, 1983, approximately 19 months from the beginning of my Geth-semane, is the day I declare I came out of isolation. I cried with joy, ''I am free!'' For that night Jean-Pierre, Amy and I attended a live theater produc-tion with 1000 people in the audience and *nothing happened.* My feelings are summed up here:

Going out tonight helped a lot, that is, the household stress I was under. The show, the loving, the touching — it helped to renew me. I've been deprived of almost everything life offers. At times, I feel close to cracking. As long as I don't think, I'm okay. I break down and cry at everything, especially scenes depicting hope or tragedy. I break down and cry with everything I touch, or eat, or breathe, and *nothing happens*. The tears are of joy.

Touching, the one human need denied us, touching — the possibility of being touched and hugged again by people, recycled in my brain — and I cried.

Touch, was the reason I'd kept Jean-Pierre in my life so long, for without his physically touching me from time to time, I would have surely died. Touch is so needed by the seriously ill and forbidden with E.I., for every touch can bring with it the spectre of death. Fear becomes one's bedmate. One cannot describe the wonder of coming out of this dark cavern into the light. What others take for granted, we take humbly and gratefully. That is the way it is.

Many new things began entering my life all at once, both positive and negative. Mostly positive. Along with my removal from isolation, I experienced severe burning pain shooting through my right eye. Unable to reach Cort in San Francisco, I began a search for an opthalmologist's office I could "survive" in. Optic neuritis is a side effect of nystatin. This terrifying symptom taught me to reduce nystatin further.

The good things more than balanced life out: ate pear — no rection, two bagels, same; started Vitamin E — no reaction; began losing some of the thirty pounds I'd put on; ate vegetables from a regular store — no reaction, children using regular shampoo — no reaction, on lower doses of nystatin (gr 1/32) and increased taheebo one ounce — felt fine.

Norman Cousins who works at UCLA heard of my miraculous recovery through a mutual friend and agreed to see me. A man lit up like a Christmas tree, he listened wholeheartedly to my nervous presentation of my particular hydrocarbon poisoning. He'd had the same, yet it took a different, but also fatal course in his body, and he had fully recovered. Norman thanked me for sharing my story and wished me the best in my desire to help the others as I got better. His visit made my whole day.

The gifts kept coming. As insignificant as the following accounts may seem, to the sufferer of candidiasis, the living death, they are miraculous.

Tuesday, May 3, I wore a brand new cotton, light blue dress with tiny white stars without washing it first in baking soda to release the formaldehyde! After wearing essentially one plaid, cotton blouse and jeans for over a year til they shredded, this was sheer heaven. I looked lovely, feeling extremely feminine and human for the first time in almost two years. I sprinted along the usual Palisadean walk. My spirit was one with the birds, bugs and flowers. Whole and peaceful, I expressed my gratitude to my Creator.

Later on that day, I was able to sort all my mail: bills, investments, notices, letters from friends, metaphysical and physical information. At last you could see my bedroom floor (my desk) again. *That in itself was a miracle!* That night, I slept for many hours, a peaceful rest, for even positive stress is exhausting when you've been ill and isolated for such a long time.

On May 16, I exclaimed again "It's over, it's over." The isolation is ended. For I went to movies three nights in a row (once a month or not at all was my previous record). Roller skated outdoors two hours on Saturday. Ate in packed Chinese restaurant. Shopped all day in department stores. Visited outdoors with friend wearing aftershave — slight tightness in chest only. At this time, I was able to add Vitamin A to my supplements.

Recovery was progressing rapidly now. So rapidly, I began believing I was totally normal again and began pushing foods once more. How I missed fruit! I tried a Mexican organic pineapple. Depression appeared at 3pm. Too soon.

Simultaneously, recovery was occurring in my relationship with Jean-Pierre. For my attitude was changing toward him. This is how I saw it:

My heart is so sad, that the tears feel ready to burst from me. When I saw Jean-Pierre tonight, I came home very saddened. Don't know if I want to cry for myself, or him, or both of us. He looks thin and pathetic, self-pitying as usual. I turn cold when he is into that for he has no reason — he's just so terribly immature, he can barely survive out there. He needs a mother and said so tonight. For once, I felt no sexual attraction for him. As I was leaving, he asked to see me Saturday night. No. *No longer interested.* Keep remembering how each time turns out anymore — crappy.

Seeing him was a constant reminder of my vulnerable state. All I want to do is cry for me, whom I've never cried for.

I was getting better.

And so a chapter of my life closes with this entry. By May 14, 1983, Saturday, I realized my isolation had truly come to an end, for it continued past my initial writing of this fact. Nineteen months of the most abject despair and indescribable joy have gone their way. It's over. The rollerskating on Venice beach for two hours — a feat I'd been unable to perform due to two major health problems — back surgery and candidiasis. Jean-Pierre and I took in all the strange sights — the disheveled, emaciated, white bearded man who preached the "religion of f..k"; a sword swallower; a mime, following fully knowing pedestrians, mimicking their person; a woman punker with bright red hair. And on and on.

Tears stream down my face at this writing — Jean-Pierre and I — a love affair gone awry. Only meant for a little while. All the pain of the past two years is over. Somehow it felt as if it would never end. This man loved me as best he could; he just wasn't for me: time revealed that to both of us. The answer is painful but true — we weren't meant for one another. I am so sad for both of us. Over and over I repeat these words. Ours was a little child love. I grew up; he stayed the same: a love loved and gone. A part of me still loves him; another knows you can love someone and not be able to live with them. I rest my case.

Every day, Eve and I found new information. Peko had recommended a book on detoxification, "Is There Any Sick Among You?" by La Dean Griffin. We learned that colonics were very useful in removing the toxins released by the Candida die-off, thereby preventing them from being reabsorbed into the intestinal tract which results in an exacerbation of symptoms, particularly fatigue. I highly recommend reading this book, bearing in mind her ideas are limited to normal detoxification. Candida defies everything known by the medical world, in fact, the Candida patient's body tends to react the opposite of all orthodox treatments. I refer specifically to routine drug therapy.

We modified Ms. Griffin's knowledge to our understanding of Candida. Eve had experimented with placing one cup of taheebo (same preparation as orally) in two quarts of colonic water. She discovered this method killed candida on contact. If she could do it, I'd try it.

A bit scared, I tried plain tap water first. Some pieces of mucus were released. Next I tried the Pau D'arco. Large amounts of mucus were expelled. I was noticeably exhausted afterwards. Being cautious with anything new, I decided the right dose of Pau for me was what I was able to take by mouth. Three ounces was my tolerance. The candida die-off was so intense in this manner that I felt very weak and faint initially. So I took two or more alfalfa tablets per hour which straightened me right out. The Pau in colonics (done no closer than three days apart) really cleared out the morning headaches, listlessness and fatigue. I also tried plain water when my abdomen swelled with gas. The rinsing broke up flatus and released trapped gas. In my case, it also alleviated the shoulder pain caused by either the nystatin or the die-off. Most of all, the colonics rapidly healed my battered body.

June passed quickly for I was busy employing colonics, reducing nystatin, letting go of Jean-Pierre, and enjoying life. There's a temptation at this stage of recovery to overdo everything. I did. So elated was I to be able to be part of life again that I tried foods, fun, and work all at once. In fact, I thought I could eat anything. Wrong. After enjoying a scoop of Haagen-Dazs ice cream and chinese food one Saturday night, I went through ''drinking'' symptoms again for three days. *Not worth it.* I also tried going into toxic buildings too fast. Accidently, I was exposed to fresh paint for about 15 minutes. Oxygen and two immunplex relieved my viselike chest pain which was followed by chills and nausea.

Another phenomenon happens too when you O.D. on Pau D'arco — you can't sleep at night. This was relieved by calcium and an immunplex. It's reassuring to know one can always be relieved of the symptoms through these means. When I was sicker, I had nothing, hence I stayed up all night suffering.

Vulnerability, both physically and mentally, occurred everytime I reduced the nystatin. I found it was very important at these times to protect myself by keeping my chemical exposure at a minimum.

Per chance, I was also put in touch with the Cancer Control Center, a non-profit organization in L.A., dedicated to researching and applying nutritional methods to healing any degenerative disease, particularly cancer. While searching for Koch's book, UCLA had referred me to this organization. On the phone, I told their Vice President my story. ''Come on down and testify at our annual convention in July.

''But I don't have cancer'' I retorted.''

''That's okay. We take anyone who has survived a fatal illness.''

I agreed to speak, though terrified of going into a hotel for any length of time. Hotels are walking chemical factories.

In any event, I'd convinced myself I was really well. This invitation gave me another shot in the arm. In fact, I felt so well I added another ounce of Pau D'arco. I still harbored the belief that, one day, I'd be able to drink four cups just like Eve, and recover faster. *Not so.* On four jiggers, exhaustion set in. Finally, I deduced, my three ounces was equivalent to Eve's four cups. That was that.

Despite going down on my dose of nystatin, the severe pain continued in my right eye. Being an ex-medical person I thought too much scaring myself out of my wits. Plus I didn't have a physician.

For in L.A. I'd been unable to find anyone who could handle a severe case. The HEAL chapter's president recommended a psychologist-turned-acupuncturist who might know something about candidiasis., When I reached him, I told him all I wanted was a physical plus immune and liver tests. He agreed. I recommended Dr. Truss's book to him, ''The Missing Diagnosis,'' to enlighten him further. He thanked me then went off to read it. As a result of his reading the book, he recognized candida in patients whose cases had puzzled him (and many other physicians) up til that time. He was really grateful to me.

The exam revealed a mild retinitis in my right eye. This scared me — I had to get off nystatin. Cort had told me this only happened on high doses over a long period of time. Well, it happened to me on gr 1/16. I had to find an opthalmologist pronto!

Meanwhile, an E.I. sufferer wrote me from Minnesota very excited about a light called the KIVA process. This lady lived in total isolation, fighting daily for her life, unable to tolerate Pau D'arco but using some nystatin. Her enthusiasm was contagious.

The letter didn't explain enough, so I decided to call her. Marge was truly happy to hear from me as she had read my articles of recovery in the Environmental Illness Association (E.I.A.) newsletter. (Strangers become instant friends in this disorder.) ''It's a four-foot fluorescent light you put in your kitchen over your food and water. Somehow it changes them from positive ions to negative ones.'' Negative ions — the natural healer? Now *I was* enthused. ''Where do I find this thing?'' ''The man producing it is Orie Bachechi.''

I phoned him immediately. Within five minutes of conversation I knew this man was on to something. Intuition told me he was the answer to my prayers. We chatted and chatted for at least an hour. He spoke physics. I understood, as I'd been studying Kriya Yoga by mail which teaches the use of the electromagnetic vibrations in healing. We comprehended one another. Now I was more excited than Marge. Without delay I ordered two lights. This was the most thrilling news to date. I'd found an answer for myself and the others who were too ill to take anything. A true blessing.

Orie knew all about acid-alkaline base in the body. But no one was familiar with candida except Eve and I who were conquering it ourselves. Orie, an amicable, natural inventor, Thomas-Alva-Edison-type, had treated a few candida cases but did not realize the suffering they were going through. He described one woman who he'd followed for a year while she used the light who'd crawled into fetal position on the floor of his office, crying incessantly, and extremely suicidal. ''That is too fast detox,'' I told him gently. ''A person could commit suicide going that fast. Too many already had for whom there was no help but we don't want to induce this suffering unnecessarily.''

Orie listened to me, telling me he'd like to work with me. From then on, he referred candida cases to me who needed the benefit of my experience. I figured out taheebo and the light had similar effects on the body — a regeneration of the immune system. How this was accomplished remained a mystery to all of us. Orie believed the light activated the pineal gland, the mysterious body at the roof of the third ventricle in the brain; he felt it activated the immune system.

Life went on while I waited for the KIVA light to arrive. Meanwhile, a big event took place in my life — I accepted an invitation to go to the premiere of the Royal Danish Ballet. Excitedly, I sent the check, then phoned the theater with my usual seemingly-crazy-questions-to-an-outsider concerning the condition of the theater. New paint? Sprayed pesticides? Recently renovated?

A sympathetic soul answered. She told me to come on over and walk through the theater the day before the ballet. (In re-entry, it's very necessary to call ahead to wherever one is going to prepare oneself for any serious chemical problems.)

With trepidation, and severe fear (an emotional complication of surviving this illness and its isolation) I drove to the theater in Beverly Hills two days before the performance. No pesticides would be sprayed. Fresh paint in a small portion of the upstairs balcony, but away from the reception area. The stage seemed the only problem. ''Usually,'' the lady told me ''they paint the stage black the night before a performance.'' Fear gripped me. *No, not paint, closed in where it had no way to ''gas out''. I couldn't survive. That well, I wasn't.* Anaphylaxis still plagued me. ''Call us back the day before. We'll know then.'' Compassion graced her voice.

Quaking inside, the phone call was made by me on June 23 . . . Lo and behold — the company was bringing its own stage. I could go. Hooray! The joy of dressing up in my sexy, black rayon dress to attend a benefit performance at a theater was the highlight of the year to date! But I wasn't that intrepid to go alone. No, I took my two bodyguards — Amy and Jen — just in case I collapsed from some substance. They knew to get me out of there, give me immunplex and oxygen.

Oxygen in tow, we went. All was well. This was Amy's first live stage show. Her black-brown eyes were huge watching the live ballet. Jen busied herself watching the pianist. He interested her, for she played the piano by ear. The reception afterwards proved successful. Amazingly, we were able to stay in spite of cigarette smoking throughout the upper balcony. Amy was bored after 3 Norwegian sodas and hor d'oeuvres, most of which she dropped on the floor. The night was a grand success in re-entry.

If June was exciting, July took a better turn. The Cancer Control Convention was July 4th weekend. I attended the first day, giving testimony to my healing. People were shocked when I told my story from the stage, and sympathetic. I spoke for only two minutes, yet was met with an avalanche of inquiries afterwards — from doctors, exhibitors and ordinary people. A minister, a healer, wanted to talk to me. A documentary film maker offered to film my story. A medical researcher asked for information on Pau D'arco. And finally, a medical science writer who was enthralled with my bizarre horror story, questioned me on the side effects of nystatin.

All in all, this was very overwhelming for a person who'd been virtually in solitary confinement while critically ill for nineteen months and slowly rejoining the world. However, the love, warmth, support and compassion of the people at the convention were so marvelous that I forgot momentarily all I'd been through. That is pretty hard to do. The recognition of my illness as valid physically, healed me even more because for once, I didn't have to explain myself.

One after the other, people came up to me. I have that . . . . I know a woman who lives in a tree house in the middle of nowhere . . . allergic to everything . . . . my wife has what you described . . . . my child and on and on. People were desperate for help. No one knew what they had. Everything the doctor's tried made them sicker. Believe me, I was no longer alone. The convention sparked my desire to write this book; the world needed it.

The only reaction I encountered that day happened when I first arrived at the hotel and sat under the air-conditioning blowers: chills, blue nails, and poor color. Twenty minutes of oxygen, which I carried in my car, straightened me out along with two immunplex. Always curious, my reaction sparked off more research. Sadly, I pin-pointed the culprit through medical reporters. Scientists at the Center for Disease Control had found the deaths from Legionnaire's disease had been caused by an organism released from the hotel's central air-conditioning system. To prevent further deaths, heavy chemicals were placed in the water tanks on top of the buildings to kill bacteria and viruses. *Voila* — chemical reactions.

My story so interested the founders of the Society that they invited me to the physicians' symposium on Tuesday. "Great! I'll try to make it." The exposure to so much at once exhausted me — even the exhilaration was too much. When I got home, I was flying high then collapsed into a dead sleep.

On July 5, the President of the Society called on me when the question was raised if anyone knew about environmental allergies. Seemed I was the only one participating in this group of fifty who had an answer. Shaky and nervous, for I'd never spoken clinically in public, I shared what I knew for 15 minutes. Many questions were thrown at me as a result. *Was the immune system damaged first? Why didn't you take amino acids?* Can't. *Why?* Shock. One doctor from Oregon knew the positive effect of taheebo on candida. He backed my story. The convention had brought me friends. Again, I was deluged by attendees at the lunch break.

"Tell your story, go to the newspapers."

"I have, they won't print it."

"Give us your name."

"Can we phone you for help?"

"Yes," I said, feeling a bit like I was on Eyewitness News with a Nobel Prize winning discovery. Really, it was all quite awesome and overpowering for me.

Brenda, my friend since March with another devastating auto-immune disease, cheered when I shared being able to be there at all. We laughed ourselves silly planning my new career as lecturer and writer on candidiasis. Somewhere, deep down inside, I knew this was my mission — to help the rest who were breaking down before they reached my stage.

But first I had to become well myself. Back to my old regime — candida diet, supplements, nystatin, Pau d'arco. Patiently I waited for the KIVA light to arrive. In the interim, I tried a bagel, my new fix. Bagels have yeast and sugar. I believed I was well enough to eat one. No. No. I felt badly the entire next day.

Los Angeles was now into her heavy smog season. Chemicals and brush-fire smoke filled the air. Not knowing which did what, I resolved to pass on bagels. By late afternoon, the head pressure was sufficient to immobilize me. Miserable, I resorted to phoning Jean-Pierre, then wished I hadn't. He rejected me out of hand. Diplomatically, I got off the phone.

When I'm in this much pain I don't want to talk to anybody, i.e. with the exception of people who are familiar with my condition. So I phoned Steve Levine in San Francisco. He loves talking to me and said he'd like to discuss our mutual experiences when he visited L.A. on the 30th. His phone calls always lifted my spirits. Yet, I also realized, I was moving too fast again.

Jean-Pierre brought foods on Saturday night as tokens of affection and forgiveness for not coming over the night before when I couldn't move my head because the nausea and pressure were so bad. He tried to be affectionate with me but the pain and stress had been too much for me. I lashed out at him viciously, raving at him for his crummy actions. As the sickening rage spewed from my mouth, twisting nausea curled my viscera. I feared ''snapping'' one more time.

But I didn't. Jean-Pierre held me in his arms as suddenly I vented my rage at my dead mother and also my rage at losing her. (She had dropped dead 3 years earlier.) ''I miss her and want her and cry out for her. I loved her very much despite her failings.'' This burst of anger cleared my vision concerning Jean-Pierre for he was like her in many ways. — *I could forgive him.* Passive, dependent, confused, sometimes kind, warm, tender Jean-Pierre, who runs from the truth. The night ended tenderly.

Ordinary minor events become major catastrophes with candidiasis. On July 19th, I collapsed from a small fire Amy accidently set in the kitchen. Semi-conscious, I fled to Jean-Pierre's. He'd used tile glue *and* sprayed pesticides for a bug that day. Thinking I was well (I *had* said this several times), he told me to come in. Now I had severe chest pain on top of collapse. He felt badly and pursued me back to my house as I stubbornly drove off in my car. Total collapse hit me in the smoky house. Again felt I was going. Amy was terrified. The whole ''family'' dumped me in the car and drove me to the Palisades. Two and a half hours later we returned. The house was cleared of smoke. Once more, I'd survived.

Still no KIVA light. Orie said the last three shipments arrived smashed. He was on top of it. Somehow July was, inconspicuously, almost gone. More puzzling events showed up. When I went out to go the bank, I felt faint and dizzy. The healer showed up that day, but I felt worse by the minute. He began a healing on me and I collapsed completely as I felt a bolt of energy flow between my eyebrows down through my body. Fear prevented me from trusting anyone by now with my health. His method was unknown to me and even scarier. I told him to get oxygen on me. Immunplex and gallons of water later, I realized I'd taken an excessive amount of Pau D'arco. The night before I'd been awake til 5am. When I did sleep, the phone awakened me at 9:30am. Now exhaustion was setting in rapidly. Smog was extremely bad that day. In that shape, the healer left me. An attempt to pick up organic food a while later worsened my condition.

The feeling of dying was upon me again . . . . Fading . . . . Panic stricken . . . . I lay on my bed. Brenda called. I could barely speak. Friend that she is, she came right over and stayed with me. She watched my hands turn yellow, my nails blue — old toxic reactions I hadn't had in a year. *I was scared.* Having her there helped my emotional state tremendously. *A real friend.* Shortly thereafter I did feel much better. In fact, I felt great and wide awake again. The healer had said I'd have a wonderful night's sleep. What he didn't know was that I'd be awake and energetic until 2am, quieting myself with readings from the Bible. Spent at last, I turned over and slept like a baby.

Brenda was gone when I awoke. I felt wonderful. Believe it or not, after all this mishap, I got gabbing on the phone and forgot about the eggs I was boiling downstairs — boiled right down to burning. Smoke was throughout the house again! In a flash, I got out. My chest and head tightened. However, the symptoms dissipated rapidly in the fresh outside air. Once again, I was grateful.

July 27, I naughtily ate homemade cookies. No reaction. Good! Currently, the Pau's healing effects were re-creating, for a second time, my old sciatic symptoms from 1976 but in a milder, transient form. Probably was caused by my increasing the tea's dose to between 7 and 10 ounces per day in an effort to balance out decreasing the morning dose only of nystatin to gr 1/32. Just didn't want to go through nystatin withdrawal again or candida rebounding against no opponent, thereby re-engendering the original symptoms. Working in the dark as I was, this strategy seemed reasonable enough to me. Plus a new wonderful development had occurred — I ate a tomato and some fruit without developing fever blisters, bleeding gums, and headaches. This absence of reactions really encouraged me to continue even more ferociously than before.

And last but not least, I was able to join Jean-Pierre in an outing to Westwood. Hundreds of nighttime denizens clogged the streets. We ventured into music stores, book emporiums and a way-out department store called *Aahs* — no ill effects. July *almost* ended on a glorious note.

Friday (July 29) dizziness, faintness, and turning yellow appeared out of nowhere. Brenda rushed over again. Sugar reaction? Could this be a delayed reaction to the cookies I ate on Monday? If this was true, I was incredibly better, for without fail this would have happened within minutes after ingesting the cookies. *No sugar*, I told myself. *You are a recovering alcoholic and sugar is what alcohol metabolizes into in the body.* At 11pm the reaction passed. The recovery was becoming faster and faster.

August was a monstrous month. On the 2nd, I tried buckwheat. By nighttime, all the symptoms of *delirium tremens* were upon me: agitation, peripheral hallucinations, crying uncontrollably about my tragic childhood, and severe paranoia. *I wanted to die.* Jean-Pierre, who'd slept over that night, was awakened at 3:30am by my restlessness. I told him I feared I would do something to myself. At the same time, I saw flashing bright yellow light throughout the room while my intestines were on fire. Metal smell in my nose — toxic reaction.

I'd also been exposed to diesel pesticides (at the Palisades), and tar fumes that day. The only thing Jean-Pierre could do was hold on to me so I didn't commit suicide. But this was only the beginning. Exposures went from bad to worse.

On August 6, I was exposed to gas cooking fumes and glue at Jean-Pierre's. Screaming at him for his stupidity (again), I ran out of his house. Chest pain, shaking chills, fighting with him. Exhausted from the strain. At home — oxygen, air conditioning and immunplex.

That same day brought 100° temperature with 90-98° humidity, and second stage smog alerts. Some brilliant neighbor decided to paint the outside of her house in this ghastly heat wave. Unfortunately for me, I didn't see her doing this til it was too late. Only outdoors briefly, my face turned red. Mental confusion descended and my mind "shattering" (the feeling of one's mind fragmenting into a thousand pieces) as an anesthetic affect crawled up my arms. Legs numb, slurred speech, crying, exhaustion.

Brenda over a third time. Three immunplexes, oxygen, lots of water. The reaction passed in two and a half hours. In fact my body became so sensitized temporarily that Brenda had to wash her hair three times with my unscented shampoo before she was "safe" to enter the room with me. Her shampoo was giving me arm and chest pain. That is a friend!

And that is progress, for if you recall what took place earlier, you will realize how far I had come. I do believe this intense sensitivity was triggered off by the buckwheat. In my experience I've found the food one eats is *extremely* important, for the ingesting of a sensitive food depresses the immune system leaving the person wide open to chemical reactions. A very valuable lesson.

My diary of August 6 summarizes the despair I was undergoing over my situation in life:

> Today, the dehumanization of my disease hit home. Once again, felled by paint fumes, I experienced severe poisoning symptoms. Helplessness, feeling of fading, dying. Horrible, nightmarish. Unreal, unbelievable, couldn't help myself.
>
> I'm realizing every ordinary human function has become a major problem: sanitary pads poisonous from added chemicals, toilet paper perfumed causing insane brain reactions, shampoo with its chest and arm pain, complete with insanity. Perfumed detergents — insanity. Petrochemicals in everything we use on a daily basis. Horrid all of it. Horrid. Beyond human comprehension. Down on my knees again asking for God's help.

I was heard. The following morning I awakened feeling just fine. Nonetheless, the severe weather continued. Earlier that year, I'd registered for a world-wide meeting of members of a meditation group. Today would be my first trip on L.A.'s freeways in two years! *I did it!* Overcoming my fear of blacking out, I drove solo with filter to the Biltmore hotel in downtown L.A. for the convocation. Whoopee! The Biltmore was unbearably stuffy and the meeting was in a sub, sub-basement. Feeling faint, I barely made it out the door before I passed out. The main point is — I was able to drive the freeway without incident — that was enough for me. For I'd blacked out at the wheel too many times while driving on them. (I don't think I need to explain the density of hydrocarbon fumes on the freeway.)

The stressful events so far this month had led me to dismiss Jean-Pierre again . . . . which brought on a dreadful loneliness. I cried copiously

— what else could I do? To be critically ill and alone is the worst fate in the world.

However, the good part is the loneliness drove me to write letters. Anything to have some contact with the human race. Since toxicity to print was gone, I wrote to anyone who would hear me. I praised Shirley MacLaine for her new book, ''Out on a Limb''; sent information to the E.I. Association newsletter regarding recovery; wrote to fellow suffers also isolated; wrote to politicians and the Environmental Protection Agency (E.P.A.); answered a letter from an E.I. who said she was well and lived 2 miles away, and a person named Chris, who couldn't use soap; I wrote my story for a magazine article; I began a book.

One blessing in August was my children's annual summer vacation with their father. Although I loved them dearly and would miss them terribly, they desperately needed a break from this ordeal before they cracked.

The heat wave continued into mid-August. I hit another ''healing crisis'' during this period which was quite a bit milder than the former ones. Once it was over, I ventured out to try going to a restaurant with my friend and financial advisor, Bill Barnard, and his co-workers. Terribly nervous, I joined the small group on Tuesday evening at a local hotel. Spotting candles on the tables, I freaked. Bill saw my fear and soothed me. ''If you can't stay, you can't stay. I'll see that you get taken care of.'' *Thanks Bill.* So I did it. Two hours in the hotel restaurant, without any reactions (even from two cigarettes), other than some pressure in my chest.

The visit was so emotionally taxing, I went home and stuffed on bagels.

August 12 loneliness struck again. I felt I'd die of it! So I called the E.I. hotline in Berkeley pouring my heart out to a kind soul named Bob. Assuaged, the deep loneliness left me and gave me strength — I was able to go on.

The children returned on August 15, just as my loneliness reached another nadir that I hardly thought I'd survive, — I'd been in so much emotional pain over letting Jean-Pierre go. But, I reasoned, for the 100th time, I must for both our sakes. For the relationship was presently so mutually destructive that any love we'd had was gone.

When Jean-Pierre received my farewell letter, lovingly saying goodbye, he called me claiming suffocation from the air to borrow my air machine. Momentarily, Jean-Pierre was back in my life again. Somehow, we wound up making lustful love. Pleasure. I needed some earthly pleasure in my life. It's abnormal to be cut off from so much the way I am, I reassured myself. That's it. I had to find ways to bring pleasure into my life besides my sporadic episodes with Jean-Pierre. But I was still too ill to date. A dilemma, a tough dilemma.

That same day, gray mucous poured from my eyes along with stabbing pain in my left jaw and ear. Recalling Eve's words, *your body will heal in reverse, as if you were running a tape of your life backwards*, reassured me. This was the return of TMJ (temporal mandibular jaw syndrome) characterized by clicking in the joint and accompanied by severe pain. Joint symptoms hounded me throughout my life since I'd had rheumatic fever at age 7. *TMJ — hm — that occurred in my twenties.* Am I that far back in my healing? I hoped so. The gray mucus was the last symptom I'd had just as I broke down completely. My body was really cleaning out.

At the same time, I felt physically changed inside. The suffering physically and emotionally the past three weeks had been exhausting but that day I felt wonderful and peaceful. Several days earlier, I'd fallen on my bed crying, begging Christ to take over and free me from my need for Jean-Pierre. For my deep need to have a man care for me when I was ill was a very strong component of my emotional tapestry. And something changed that day. I lay in bed three nights, wide awake till 2 or 3am, serene and feeling whole. Awesome — unexplained, but true. Furthermore, no more symptoms of the disease existed, save a slight numbness in my hands around after-shave. No cerebrals. So confident was I that I was totally healed, (once more), I discontinued nystatin and Pau D'arco on the 23rd. Just didn't feel I needed it anymore.

On the 24th, I woke up with severe soreness surrounding my breasts and breastbone — a bruised feeling. This sensation was like the previous week when my liver area was sore. My kidney area was also feeling very bruised. Peculiar feeling I was being cleansed of toxins. The thymus gland is located in the breastbone. My body felt totally different. I speculated that the thymus was activated that day (presently believed by physicians to be the initiator of the immune system). The taheebo was doing its job well.

Elated by my inner metamorphesis, my high energy, and my healthy feelings, I changed the locks on my doors. Finally, *really* letting go of Jean.-Pierre I convinced myself that now I was entirely well.

This delusion was destroyed on August 26. Feeling extremely well, I shopped at a local natural foodstore. As I walked towards the back, I smelled fresh pesticides. Thinking nothing could happen to me I kept right on shopping. My overconfidence nearly cost me my life.

Suddenly, blotchy red spots appeared all over my face, followed by numbness and generalized weakness. My newly hired nurse's aide rushed me home. Dinah had worked for me before when I had back problems, so I was relieved to be in familiar hands. The usual — immunplex, oxygen. Plus two new items — bee pollen and licorice root tea (adrenal supporter).

My skin became yellow tinged. The aide, not understanding the seriousness of what had happened, kept asking me questions. Blurredly, I told her to leave me be. Was she blind? Couldn't she see my color? Obviously she could handle backs but not this.

Around 5pm, I felt better . . . . Watery orange-brown diarrhea . . . . Ate some food with a dash of cayenne to relieve the vasculitis. Decided walking would help. At the Palisades . . . . a brown streak of L.A.'s famous pollution rose above the ocean . . . . a brush fire was burning . . . . Inhaled smoke . . . . weak, confused, nausea . . . . home . . . . more licorice tea . . . . phoned Peko . . . . ''Try a mixture of ginger, cayenne and olive oil to help you . . . . Liver detoxifiers . . . .

I'd forgotten my own rule of thumb — *never cut nystatin.* Withdrawal had left my body extremely vulnerable. Peko suggested going off nystatin a small dose at a time, every other day while supplementing the void with kantita and chemex herbs, (a new non-toxic herbal formula discovery designed to assist E.I. sufferers), rather than abruptly stopping it. Her idea made sense. I took one dose, gr 1/32, of nystatin that evening, (presently, I'd been weaning myself from nystatin since last May — 3 months) and ordered the herbs.

The following entry, as incredible as it seems, actually befell me:

August 28,   Exposed to bad chemical yesterday (pesticides?) while I was sitting in my bedroom with the windows open in late afternoon. The smell poured into my house. Viselike . . . . chest pain . . . . Cried out to girls — ''Get the oxygen, close the windows, turn on the filters — we have to get out of here'' . . . . We fled in my car, where I sat bent over the wheel gasping for air . . . . Just like a heart attack! Several hours later we re-entered the house. Tried concoction of herbs — parsley, comfrey, mullein, black walnut and licorice root . . . . Severe diarrhea afterwards . . . . Cleansed out my system . . . .

10:30 *that night* — Walked outside on patio. More pesticides! God .... it! Slight chest symptoms. Used cayenne — worked! Shaking chills . . . . called therapist . . . . Took immunplex . . . .

August 29,   Woke up feeling as if I'd die . . . . Severe diarrhea, with tons of water past 3 days . . . . Color yellow on and off . . . . Throat and lungs burning, severe nausea . . . . called my doctor . . . . Went to office collapsed from toxic building . . . . cold sweats . . . . Doctor phoned Dr. Cort in San Francisco . . . . ''Don't touch her! Get someone to get her down to the ocean for fresh air — it will clear her lungs'' . . . . Demanded doctor draw liver enzymes and pesticide poisoning test . . . . He drew the first; the latter he contacted a doctor in New Orleans, a poisoning specialist. He never phoned back . . . . Met Dr. Luc, an M.D., acupuncturist. He performed acupressure on certain meridians . . . . Miraculously, my head cleared! I began to feel better. Back home. Nurse's aide and Brenda helping. Brenda went to the neighbors telling them I was seriously ill because someone had sprayed pesticides on the outside shrubbery. No one admitted doing it, even though you could smell the pesticides all over the outside!

Day of sheer anxiety that I'd die.

Haven't been this way since Berkeley when I first broke down . . . . Color pale to yellow tinge . . . . Scariest day I've had since I don't know when . . . .

August 31. Rough, rough day . . . . Down, so down . . . . crying on and off all day . . . . Despair . . . . Weak . . . . Worn out . . . . Called Hotline in Berkeley — no help . . . . Cried most of time . . . . Took walk and talked to God . . . . Asked him to take me — end this pain . . . . I have nothing left to lose . . . . Cried on the phone to Brenda . . . .

The worst was over. I believe the herbs and Dr. Luc saved my life. And God. Night sweats continued (in air conditioning). Lost about ten pounds. Listlessness, apathy, and depression continued into the first week of September. When I saw Dr. Luc on September 6, he said my immune system was way down. Acupressure helped somewhat. From Luc, I learned another way of viewing the body. His knowledge coincided with my study of energy fields. This physician was the first professional whom I encountered, who'd brought me a light at the end of this dark tunnel. He agreed to add his knowledge to this book.

Luc was interviewed by phone at his home in the San Fernando valley where he was babysitting his 2 and 4 year old children:

What is your background?

I received my M.D. in Belgium in '71 and my doctor of acupuncture in '81, after three years of study in Paris.

How do you define Candidiasis?

Candidiasis, according to acupuncture, is spleen deficiency, a loss of energy to that organ. The spleen is considered the ''Mother of all organs'' by the Chinese. The immune system and the spleen are connected. The liver controls the spleen. When the liver has more control (too much energy) the spleen becomes deficient. As a result, the overenergized liver will produce angry outbursts out of nowhere. Alcohol, for example, is a chemical which overheats the liver causing damage. In acupuncture, too much energy to an organ is the ''yang'' or negative energy.

What is the etiology of E.I.?

Heriditary factors play a large role. Patients come in to me telling me there were other family members with outburst of violence, anger, or extreme irritability unrelated to what is transpiring in life.

Food substances bring on spleen deficiency. Raw and cold foods, salads in particular, drain the spleen's energy. The stomach and spleen are the same entity transforming and transporting food through the spleen. Too much of these foods decreases the spleen's ability to 50% of normal which produces a myriad of symptoms: morning diarrhea, fatigue, cerebral fatigue — memory disturbances, loss of concentration, spaciness, fogged brain, abdominal distortion, gas, bloating feeling after eating, to name the major ones. The body attempts to react to excessive heat by producing more heat. Prolonged hyper-energizing of the body produces stagnation of function taking the body from constant heat to the other extreme, constant cold. These people who are cold all the time, who have gone from yang energy (negative) to all yin (positive), have the worst prognosis and take longer to return to health.

Climate — Dampness (molds) are the biggest enemy of the spleen. No one should live in damp climates, but especially candidiasis patients for it beings the spleen down. Hyperventilation, caused by the depression of the spleen can cause respiratory alkalosis. PCO_2 (arterial blood gas) drains enormous amounts of energy leaving the patient helpless and unable to move. Total exhaustion sets in. Person feels as if she is dying, but usually she won't, unless the drainage is continuous. Dampness is the worst climate factor. Heat does not cause this degree of adverse reactions in the body. I recommend a dry, moderate environment for healing. Air conditioning will help in humid areas with the respiratory problems.

Exterior factors such as petrochemicals — tars, paints, and pesticides — their toxic fumes are a major factor in today's toxic world depressing the immune system breaking down the more vulnerable first, the chemically sensitive individual. Antibiotics, the pill, cortisone, immunotherapy, some anesthetics, halothane in particular which is severely liver toxic, and hair dye are a few more of the primary culprits.

Interior factors also lead to spleen deficiency. Emotions. Worry, obsessive — compulsive behavior, analytical minds — the Type A personality — depresses energy. This is not a psychiatric disorder at all, but a physical one causing mental aberrations. It's treated this way (mental) simply because it is not understood by Western medicine.

Is there a personality change?

Yes. If you bring energy down, the person becomes more and more obsessed by the past; extreme worrying develops; a regression to childhood occurs; and a negative toxic personality develops. I've seen the personality return to normal with treatment.

How would you treat candidiasis?

First, I'd balance the energy with acupuncture or acupressure. Second, proper food. Third, a change in life style. These people are caught in a vicious cycle. They live a rigid life style, which becomes more rigid as the disease progresses. They need to break away from this rigidity by changing their attitudes. I stress exercise. Walks. Move. No matter how little. It moves the toxins out of the body. Meditation will pull you out of non-cerebral reactions. And lastly love. Any love you can get anywhere is the greatest healer. Whether through a psychotherapist, friends, or a support group. You need love to heal.

Do you feel these people are "crazy" or hypochondriacs as other people see them?

No. It's multiple physical factors mainly, part of a syndrome. Totally wrong. Easy to name a hypochondriac, but incorrect.

In seeing these patients, please tell me the degree of sickness you've seen and the prognosis?

I've seen many different degrees. The smallest is manifested in menstrual disturbances, angry behavior, and fatigue. These symptoms are so common with other diseases, they are not recognized as such. The patient goes to a regular doctor and is treated only as an organ, and he misses the diagnosis. The doctor hooks the patient with a label according to his specialty.

The worst cases [however] probably can't even make it into my office, or, they wind up in hospitals and possibly, die.

Are all the cases the same breakdown?

Same evolution. Candida is the common organism overgrowing in the body.

Why are women more affected?

May not be, for more women see doctors than men and usually, take more drugs. Hormones are possible, but I don't have the experience to answer your question.

What is your opinion of nystatin?

Unfortunate side effects. It aggravates the symptoms so badly in the first week, many patients give it up because they are suffering too much. Then, the patients on nystatin for several months go through terrible withdrawal symptoms. I believe in healing the natural way. Yes, I would recommend the candida herbs and Pau D'arco. I don't believe in much medication. I have no experience with Nizerole or Amphotericin B. I believe we are just badly educated regarding the use of drugs as the only method. I need to give the patients confidence that natural methods will heal them. That's the important factor. A caring relationship with the physician. Probably heals more than any drug.

Do you recommend the candida diet?

In part. Steamed vegetables and warm food are my suggestion. Not raw or cold. Cold drinks and ice cubes deplete the spleen. Eventually when the patient is well she can eat raw foods in moderation only. Sweets belong to the spleen. One should have a small amount, preferably daily. Not sugar. Natural sweetness. Steamed green vegetables will provide energy for the spleen while it repairs itself. Otherwise, I agree with the diet.

Do you verify the critical nature of my case?

Yes. And I saw you two years into treatment, and you were still very ill with anaphylaxis.

Do you consider E.I. allergy, or toxic poisoning?

More toxic poisoning — hydrocarbon poisoning to be exact. A person with hydrocarbon allergy, e.g. headaches from perfume, vomiting around diesel fumes, is a functioning person in society which is differentiated from the seriously ill person with hydrocarbon poisoning who has an almost vegetable-like existence.

Do you believe these people can ever be totally well or return to working in toxic buildings?

I wouldn't advise them to return to toxic buildings. We need to change the toxic environment, not adjust even a healthy person, to the poisons emitted in today's buildings. The lights, carpeting, air systems etc. are making everyone sick.

Do you believe these people should be put on all types of chemicals — thyroid, progesterone etc. to "treat" the local symptoms or treat the candida first?

No local treatment. That's only symptomatic treatment. I believe, once again, we have to look at the whole person. Some need to correct one of the causative factors more than the other. The food, perhaps more than the environment. Control candida first, I agree.

In my personal experience, treating the candida, then healing the immune system, and regenerating the intestinal flora, produces a natural resumption of the functions of the affected organs. Do you agree with this observation?

Yes. Totally.

Thank you, Dr. Luc for your time and love.

Dr. Luc's theory on spleen deficiency made sense. But the mosaic was not complete — how does one regenerate the intestinal flora to begin the process? The answer was drawing closer and closer. For at long last, in my possession, were the KIVA lights, through which the final piece to this puzzle would be presented.

THE KIVA PROCESS

September has always been a month of new beginnings for me. The 6th marked the fourth anniversary of my sobriety — a feat in itself. Considering the negativity in August, September blossomed into the beginning of the end of my healing.

The light had arrived two days before the anaphylactic reactions from the pesticides commenced. When I phoned Orie he said, ''It's okay to use it — go slowly, leave it on for five minutes at first. You'll experience your symptoms again.''

No way. Being so close to death with anaphylaxis, I wasn't about to try out the light under these terrifying circumstances. After all, the light was experimental. I waited.

Meanwhile, Peko was teaching me the art of the pendulum by phone; it tested the herbs she'd rushed to me during this episode, for toxicity to my system. The pendulum is very ancient, a ball-shaped crystal on a string with which a person can determine what will or won't harm them physically. The procedure is simple: place the herb or food to be tested in one hand. Place the pendulum over the substance. Ask yourself ''Is this product . . . . good for me?'' If it is, the pendulum will swing clockwise in a circle indicating yes; otherwise it swings counter-clockwise denoting no. When this part is done you ask the pendulum if one tablet, etc., is the correct dose for that day. One repeats the entire procedure with each question.

When I'd first seen the pendulum in use a year earlier by some critically ill woman with E.I. in Marin, I freaked. *They are practicing witchcraft.* Six months later when I met Peko, she taught me how to use it. Even then, I wasn't ready to listen. No, what it took was for me to be so ill that putting any new substance in my mouth could have proved fatal. I became a believer.

The herbs she'd sent me for liver detox — bayberry and dandelion root — registered *no* on the pendulum. "That's okay," Peko reassured me, "Perhaps as you get well, you will be able to tolerate them at a future date." Peko's soft caring voice was always welcome.

The same thing happened with the KIVA light that precipitated my employing the pendulum — desperation. For up until September 9, I remained detached, crying, and depressed on a daily basis from the poisoning. I didn't even care that it marked two years of staying alive after pananaphylaxis. Jean-Pierre brought me four roses and a George Winston album to celebrate. Beautiful. Touching. Yet, I didn't care. He still loved me but my feelings for him were gone.

My hair was falling out in clumps. An intuition told me to try two more small doses of nystatin to alleviate my suffering: it helped!

On September 10, the night sweats stopped and I also stabilized on three doses (gr 1/32) of nystatin which I still needed. Dr. Luc said my kidneys had received a severe blast. The way he described anaphylaxis to me was as if an atom bomb had gone off, over and over, in my body. He too was amazed I was alive. I told him about the KIVA light. Luc was very interested, for Orie's process he agreed, was a physical manifestation of chinese acupuncture paralleling his knowledge that balancing energy in the nervous system allows the body to heal itself naturally. Acupuncture's theory is equivalent to the laws of physics. Orie knew physics. Had we discovered a new era in medicine combining the two?

The acute phase of this poisoning ended September 13. This episode proved to me that I had a ways to go to being well. The time was right for the KIVA light for the wind left my sails during this lengthy episode. The mental ravagement was the most difficult to get over. Once you're enjoying a reprieve for any length of time, a new attack can devastate you emotionally. From this I learned a great lesson — I am well for today — what will be will be. That way I could diffuse the emotional roller coaster I was on. On September 14, I began the KIVA process, which was to turn the whole disease around in three months time!

Orie had instructed me to turn on the light for five minutes in order to evaluate my reaction. In this way he could determine the level of my toxicity. Here we go!

After installing the bulbs in my ceiling fixture and removing the decorative plastic inserts (plastic interferes with the light's penetration), I switched on the light. A quiet, gentle, peacefulness came over me. "That's good," he said. Since I felt the light was equivalent to Pau D'arco in its potency, I informed Orie I'd use the light for half an hour or so, rather than the 72 hours straight he'd recommended. I also stopped Pau D'arco temporarily. At 45 minutes under the light, extreme agitation appeared. "Good" Orie declared — "That means your pineal gland is activated."

Orie also told me I could use tap water. Not believing this, I placed tap water in a glass pitcher under the light. After 30 minutes (his time allotment), the water tasted of chlorine. Disappointed, I phoned him. "The water must be extremely contaminated out there," he replied. "Yes, it is Orie, *The Citizens for a Better Environment* and other organizations have found the groundwater is poisoned throughout the state with pesticides, solvents, and other chemicals."

"Fine," Orie said. "Let's try your plastic-bottled water." Now, I can *taste* the plastic in bottles, so I considered myself an excellent judge of the truth in this area. After thirty minutes under the light, there was no taste of plastic left! *Now* I *was* convinced. Orie laughed. A wonderful partnership in healing was about to evolve.

That first day, I placed all my food and water under the light for at least 30 minutes. Orie explained he took up where John Ott left off. Ott, a photographer, had discovered different colored lights affect different plants, either negatively or positively in growth. Mr. Bachechi took his knowledge one step further, applying it to food and water. Genius, absolute genius! Never in the entire time of my recovery was I as excited about anything as this development. Intuitively, I knew this was the answer I had been searching for.

Wanting to maintain my credibility with fellow E.I.'s (many knew how ill I'd been and my miraculous recovery to date), for whom I wrote occasional articles how I was doing it, I decided to keep quiet about the light til it did what it was purported to to.

I had a few days experimenting with the light before I was scheduled to tell my story at the H.E.A.L. meeting. Maybe, I'd have even more hope for the others by then, I mused. The major changes that took place within the first week were astounding: lost large amount of toxic bloat, graying hair turning back to chestnut brown, and huge amounts of energy.

At the same time, I began switching over to the candida herbs. Nystatin alternating with the herbs worked well. Orie had told me my drug need would be cut in half very shortly. This was wonderful news as I had retinitis from nystatin which really worried me. And Orie went on, "The withdrawal symptoms will be cut way down." Every utterance from his mouth raised my spirits.

Orie and I kept in very close touch during the early days of the treatment. He gave me the name of a critically ill patient in Minnesota to talk to who was having great success with the light. We became instant phone friends.

Signs that the light was working were many. Initially my body threw off huge amounts of mucous rectally, my urine began burning (very acidy), and I went from diarrhea to passing black stools. Orie said this meant my pineal gland was activated by the light which in turn activated the thymus gland, which was the catalyst for activating the immune system to regenerate. He gave me information as I was ready for it, that is, as my symptoms brought it to my consciousness. Surely, he was on to something.

To show you how far I'd come with the light in just a few days, let me share that I was able to sit in a brand-new theater through the four-hour French silent film, ''Napoleon!'' And on September 18, my birthday, Brenda took me to a packed theater playing, ''Return of the Jedi.'' Prior to the light I'd always attended half-empty matinees where I could change my seat if someone sat near me with perfume or after shave.

By the ninth day ''on'' the light, a healing crisis began. That very same day, I was to address the local H.E.A.L. chapter regarding my inspiring recovery.

Right before my evening talk I discovered I couldn't read my notes from the pink index cards — the color was too glaring. So under an extreme time limit I began the re-write on white cards while simultaneously eating dinner and drying my hair. The phone rang continuously. Ready to scream, I kept on trucking. In the middle of all this tension Jean-Pierre showed up. I told Amy to send him away but he barged in the front door anyway. ''Will you take my watch to the jeweler's to get fixed?'', he asked blandly.

His inappropriate request enraged me. ''Leave me alone. Get the hell out of here. Can't you see I have a speech to make tonight? I need support, not demands!

''You can take my watch for me'' he reiterated blankly.

Jean-Pierre's madness was just that.

''Get out of here you idiot. I have to be ready in half an hour to speak.''

''What time is the talk?'' the zombie spoke.

''You're not invited.''

''Why not?'' he asked stupidly.

''I don't want any negative person there like you telling me what I said wrong or who I offended. I don't want you there. That's it. Now get out.''

Without responding, he left.

My goal was to help fellow sufferers; no one or nothing was going to stand in my way. Despite the added immediate stress, I'd arisen like the Phoenix out of the ashes transcending these circumstances, overcoming the residual symptoms of the pesticide poisoning to deliver my speech, proving one can overcome anything if the goal is to serve mankind. Mine was.

Praying for a reprieve from the healing crisis and with a great deal of nervousness, I drove to the lecture room in Beverly Hills. Having never been able to speak in front of a room full of people due to severe stage fright, I prayed for Jesus to speak through me just as I was announced to begin. My first public speech in my entire life flowed forth like a spring. It was easy.

The information was received with gratitude and excitement; the talk was a success. A seed had been planted — the others were given hope. Briefly I mentioned the astonishing effects of the KIVA light. One or two people really heard me. Especially a man named Tom Carmichael who'd suffered the brain toxicity of this ailment since 7 years old. He presently was 41. He approached me with tears in his eyes saying, ''You've given me hope for the first time in my life." Tears filled mine. Little did I know then, this lovely man was to become very important in my life.

By 11pm that night, the healing crisis was in full swing. Yet, with the light, it was different — less intense but more results. Orange colored stools appeared. Orange oozed from my gum line. Curious, I asked Orie if he knew what I was excreting. "That's old penicillin and sulfa. Ever have any?" "Yes, tons in childhood," I exclaimed. Concurrent to my detox, Amy developed abdominal and kidney pain followed by passing large amounts of orange-red stools. She'd been on small amounts of taheebo along with me but had fainted on one ounce. So she too had been beginning to break down. Now she was building up right along with me. Jen was very healthy but experienced mild cold symptoms. The effect of the girls eating and drinking the KIVA products was that the whole family was healing. Orie had said the light would detox the whole house. He wasn't kidding — even the pet mice became stronger (We experimented on them with the water too).

Mucus discharged from my throat and vagina. Nystatin was cut back to gr $\frac{1}{64}$; the other two doses remained at gr $\frac{1}{32}$. Changing from nystatin was tricky, so I won't go into a lot of detail here. What I will mention is that withdrawing from nystatin was easier this time around.

Plaque was falling off my lower teeth. With candidiasis heavy plaque and gingivitis are common problems. Orie had told me the light disintegrated plaque, but honestly, I was skeptical. It was true. Then food cravings returned. Peanuts, my old friend. Stuffing again.

The baking soda bath sounded like a good way to help release these toxins. The water turned murky gray. (Better in the tub than coloring my body). My body was loaded with poisons. Weakness, headache, and nausea appeared afterwards. Large green bowel movement. Orie said I was cleaning out. *I sure was.* Too fast. Slowed down again.

With the KIVA process slowing down consists of turning the light off. That simple. Nothing invasive nothing to wait for to wear off. The reaction stops when the light is not in use. Til now there had been nothing this effective or safe.

"The dramatic changes," Orie explained "occur with the light within the first ninety days." He asked if I would record the differences to prove *what* the light *did*. Gladly, I complied.

The 17th day on the light, September 29, I felt so good, I gorged on bagels — and luxuriated myself with the joy of a nectarine. Fruit had been totally out for me for two years! Along with enjoying these goodies, Dr. Luc, who performed acupressure on me that day, told me he was amazed at my recovery from the poisoning. In fact he told his associate, Dr. Milkos, who was shocked at the super-positive change in my condition. So shocked in fact that he called Orie and made plans to fly to Albuquerque to consult with him. Coincidentally, my old pre-surgery back symptoms returned in a milder form.

But the best part of all this was my girlfriend Joelyn's coming to visit me the night before to celebrate our AA and my natal birthdays. Her visit was significant. Prior to this night, we'd never been able to stay in my house together. Detergent in her clothes or a slight scent of perfume picked up on her hair traveling to my house had caused me cerebrals with chest and arm pain. *Nothing happened* when she was there. I cried with joy. The KIVA light had made it possible for me to allow people in my home again. The semi-isolation was now ending. *This in only two weeks on the light.* Gleefully, I waited for the next development.

At three weeks, my energy was endless. Throughout the first few weeks of the light I passed huge amounts of brown mucus. Colonics came in very handy here as the mucus would have been reabsorbed, making me sicker.

So well was I that On October 2, I attended a discussion by Godfrey Reggio, an ex-priest, of his controversial film, ''Koyaanisquatse'' which means in Hopi Indian language, ''Life out of Balance''. Essentially, he said we'd created a twentieth century Frankenstein and the monster — named technology — was taking us over. ''The technological girdle strangulating us all,'' he went on, ''is becoming an awareness to more and more people.'' Stimulating, so stimulating. Someone else knew what was happening besides me. I raised my hand and told Godfrey of the technology-induced immune disease in detail before a shocked audience. He wanted to know more. So I told him I'd catch him on the break. As I continued listening to Godfrey speak, I fell in love in the back of the room with him, a huge (about 6'6'') bear of a man, light brown hair, soft eyes and very humble. I fell out of love when he told me he lived in isolation with his film group and was dedicated to producing his films. Oh well.

But he did give me his address and his Italian, producer friend invited me to the showing of his film about life *in* balance. Knowing neither of them knew the extent of the horror I was speaking about, and also knowing I didn't know if I could survive the downtown movie theater, I accepted the invitation. My God, I told myself, I survived this little church auditorium filled with about five hundred people! Why not try a drive to smoggy L.A., by sidestreets, and try to go? I was elated by my freedom.

That same night, I also met a reporter from a local, radical environmental newspaper which advocated anarchy and slaughter as a means to change our leaders' minds about the need to deal with the pervasive pollution erupting everywhere. When I told him I refused to be interviewed because they advocated violence, he jumped up and down in the aisle like a madman screaming ''It will be necessary to murder others to make them see our point of view!'' His spaced, glazed eyes made me realize what a terrified soul he was. ''Right he (Reggio) was,'' I said, ''We do need change fast. Violence is not the way but educating the masses.'' Shaken, I departed from him abruptly only to be besieged by the Green Party members who were outside the front door collecting signatures to replan Santa Monica and keep out indoor pollution.

The night was enlightening. So, others are angry and awake too. Some drugged, some not. Godfrey commended me on my work with the critically ill E.I.'s, thanking me for my information. (I forgot to mention — when I could I assisted fellow sufferers by phone, mail, or articles to share the hope I was experiencing). He looked at me with soft eyes, lit up a cigarette (that definitely ended the romance), and said "Write to me, I'm very interested in your knowledge." *I will Godfrey, when the time is right.*

The detoxing continued. Orie had warned me that anything might be expelled from my system. He was right. The colon seemed to be the main avenue of escape for the materials which had been retained in my system. Most of that first month I felt my body was roto-rootering, cleaning out a veritable sewer. One does not realize what they've done unconsciously to their bodies until you start eliminating junk from your body. All the items that made you sick. "Why, one man," Orie remarked laughingly, "passed an entire sausage skin!" That's hysterical!

The third week of the program, leg and kidney pounding began — yet much less than on nystatin or Pau. I'd cut Pau out a week earlier when detox became too strenuous and used only one ounce every three days. I further reduced nystatin to two doses, gr 1/64, adding two Chemex and two Kantita spansules in their place. Again, I passed a huge amount of foul smelling black-brown diarrhea. Never had my body healed so gently nor so thoroughly. I really felt I'd be totally well very, very soon.

And on it went. Going off nystatin was the most challenging part of this new chapter. Too low — withdrawal; too high — detox. Through trial and error, I discovered reducing one dose of gr 1/32 to gr 1/64 per month, was what my metabolism could handle, interspersed with adding the herbs one more day at a time in between, til the dose just disappeared into oblivion. It was gentle, it was slow — the only way to go and not suffer.

Likewise, the suffering with Jean-Pierre followed the same path — less and less seeing him til he disappeared into never-again-land. As lonely as I was, seeing him brought about further alienation. When he invited me to go away with him for the weekend of October 14, I declined. He was so unrealistic. I barely could survive in my own house or outside. At this stage traveling to a totally new environment overwhelmed me. Sanity clearly prevailed. He is empty and needs to escape. His self-absorption and thoughtlessness would drag me down. This was too much stress for me whom had to very slowly re-enter life and was very, very anxious about it.

The relationship was so dead that we'd sit in my bedroom together, he on a chair, me in the bed, and give me multiple excuses for not making love. Somewhere along the way, I'd sadly realized he needed me sick. Getting well, being the strong, dynamic person I am was more than he could cope with.

That day I sat on my bedroom floor and cried over my human deprivation of love and touch. *So needy.* Being around Jean-Pierre had become an emotional torture chamber for me. Not that he meant to be one. Empty shells are always like this. But like I said before, every dark moment brought with it the challenge to find a new option.

The answer came through a person, an AA member who informed me that 4 new non-smoking meetings had opened in Pacific Palisades. Her call really lifted my spirits. If I could get the love and support I needed through AA, detaching from this painful situation with Jean-Pierre would be a lot easier. At present all I had to contend with was: could I survive in the buildings they were housed in? Life seemed better.

That Monday, on a planned night with Jean-Pierre, an accident occurred that changed the whole event from one of pleasure to one of fear. The house filled with smoke from a faulty toaster. Collapsed again. But no chest pain. Jean-Pierre was like a lunatic, threatening to punch Jen in the mouth as he kept shaking me telling me to give him my doctors name, and she told him ''Can't you see? My mom is almost unconscious?'' The three of them turned on filters and opened windows then dragged me to the car. A ride to the Palisades where I could inhale fresh air. The semi-conscious state passed in 2½ hours.

The next day when I saw Dr. Luc—he was *very* concerned. He treated me with accupressure which brought on a medium anaphylactic reaction. This was the first time he'd seen me dissolve into one. I fell into a chair half-conscious passing through shaking chills, and crying. Luc said he watched the color drain right out of me from the top of my head to the tips of my toes. Weeping, in a brain reaction, I told him I couldn't take anymore. Tenderly, he said, ''Elizabeth, you are much better. You recover rapidly these days. Before it was weeks. Remember that.'' Suddenly, my brain cleared up; the reaction ceased. Without Luc's compassion, I doubt I would have snapped back so easily. He gave *me* hope!

Two AA meetings went well. I celebrated my belated birthday. So overjoyed was I to have a connection back with life that I cried through my birthday speech. ''There is a God, the Steps work on everything, and a sense of humor will get you through anything'', I declared to anyone who would hear me. Old acquaintances and new hugged me — after I'd announced my restrictions that no one with after-shave or perfume was to touch me. The hugs did wonders for me. I felt at home again. A male AA member working with psychic healing for AIDS patients, asked to use my name in a newspaper article, making known to the public that taheebo and the KIVA light mended the immune system. A bit reluctantly I said yes, afraid the resulting publicity would be too much for me. The time was not right for this development.

In the middle of all this another pressure descended upon me: my roof had seventeen leaks. The rainy season began in November. The thought of using deadly chemicals to repair the roof caused me severe anxiety and nightly nightmares.

The scariest nightmare went like this: *I returned to my home at 3:30pm, to find it black inside . . . Try to turn on the lights. Won't work . . . Hear*

*someone walking upstairs . . . Try to dial friend . . . phone not work-
ing . . . finally phone rings . . . a person who looks like me comes down the
stairs from 2nd floor . . . Room is silver — luminous where figure
stands . . . an insane dog runs down the stairs (my childhood dog, Suzie),
rust-brown chihuaha-terrier with the figure . . . barking and springing thru
the air, running in continuous circles . . . a warning all's not right . . . friend
will be over . . . hang up . . . terrified alone with luminous figure, unreal,
almost statue-like in appearance . . .*

The dream appeared to be warning me (the dog) not to use the odorless
chemicals recommended by one roofer. Odorless but deadly formaldehyde!
The luminous figure I believe was a spirit telling me I'd be allright, not to fear,
that I'd be protected. A warning and a blessing simultaneously. What to do?

Again I prayed. The answer came through an honest roofer. "You don't
need the roofers. This is a job for the sheet metal man." *How simple. And
non toxic.* On my knees, I thanked my Maker.

Brenda announced she was going back home to Florida for the holidays. That night I descended into the pits of despair. I couldn't stop crying.
Her leaving and my giving up Jean-Pierre at the same time — I couldn't bear
it. They were the only two human beings who'd been close to me in my
suffering and both were leaving me at the same time. Abandonment! Even
my therapist failed to understand. She said, "She's only leaving for a month
and a half."

"A month and a half!" I raved, "When it's the only friend you have who
understands what you are going through." I wanted to rant at Zena and
Jean-Pierre too, but feared losing even their sympathetic ear. Zena finally
understood when she recalled another patient who'd lost her only friend.
*Devastated. Close, Zena, but not as horrible as being critically ill and losing
your only friend.* I needed compassion in my panic state, for the longer this
disease goes on, the more fear and alienation from people builds up. I had
reached my peak.

Jean-Pierre happened to call late that hight, so I cried and raved about
overload til midnight. He was very sympathetic, for being an emotional
isolate himself, he understood my despair. He offered to help. "Please pick
up food at the natural food store tomorrow." "Okay," he murmured softly. It
was the first time he'd offered to assist me domestically in the three plus
years I'd known him. Being desperate, I did not turn him down. For the
poisoning, roof, Brenda leaving, and losing him were so overwhelming for
me that old feelings about terror of life swept over me. Again, I prayed for
help in this situation. It came — in a very unexpected way — but that's
getting ahead of myself.

Time also was bringing life closer and closer to me every day. For
example I attended Jen's open house at the university-sized Santa Monica-
Malibu high school. To walk so many stairs and distances, to go in and out of
toxic classrooms, to confer with her teachers would have been impossible a

month ago. Jen was thrilled at my attendance, so happy indeed, she chatted endlessly with me about my reaction to her teachers.

By October 23, re-entry was in full swing bringing with it a myriad of explosive emotions. Engulfing fear anticipated every new attempt at going into my once hostile environment. To cope with these paralyzing emotions I began studying yoga breathing exercises via mail. Breathing deeply, while clearing my mind mentally, then releasing the air through deep exhalation, had a totally calming effect on my body. The oxygenation of all my cells through these methods seemed to enhance my healing both physically and mentally. I vowed to continue the practice on a limited basis (about 5-10 minutes) while my strength built up.

By the end of October, my body was strengthened sufficiently to try a stronger type of taheebo. *Strong.* Exposure to tar that same day only resulted in chest tightness — no pulmonary vasculitis. Terribly overconfident again, I binged on bagels the following Monday. Couldn't stop eating them. On Wednesday, I almost jumped out a window. *Alcoholic symptoms again.* Jean-Pierre sat with me, literally holding me down on my bed till the reaction passed at 2am. *"No more bagels, Elizabeth, please",* he implored me. Simultaneously we had a Santa Ana condition. I believe my severe response was a combination of both, for the forbidden food lowered my immune defenses while also making me more vulnerable to the winds. I say this because, when I closed the sliding glass door of my bedroom, the insanity, nausea, and headache disappeared instantaneously.

If the Santa Anas didn't prove my undoing, the next crisis did. The roofer told me he'd discovered termites nested in the wood beams where he had to nail down the sheet metal. I couldn't believe my ears. *Termites! Pests! Pesticides!* Oh Lord, no. Pesticides would kill me! What were the alternatives? Meanwhile, ominous clouds predicted an imminent rainstorm and the termites had to be destroyed before he could seal the roof. I was fighting nature all the way.

Halloween morning I put my brain back together and began making phone calls. Citizens for a Better Environment referred me to a fellow in Berkeley who researched non-toxic alternatives. He referred me to a professor at UCLA who'd invented an electron-gun to kill pests. UCLA told me he was retired. Back to Berkeley. Phone a woman in Sacramento who knew where the gun was located. Las Vegas. Reached the company's president. Explained my dilemma. Extremely cooperative. He phoned Redondo Beach, an hour's drive south of Santa Monica, to inform the only company in Southern California carrying the gun of my dilemma. They'd be out late that very afternoon.

Mr. Bondy explained to me how the gun worked. "A positive-ion charge is instilled into the wood. The electricity travels through the wooden beams, filling nests with deadly electrical current. The termites along the way are electrocuted. (And only ⅓ the price of a total fumigation, plus not destroying the people living in the house!) Great. Just great. I thanked him profusely for his care and concern promising to pass on the news to other E.I.'s.

Halloween night Jay Tallon arrived. The girls and I left our house and stood outside watching. As sensitive as my body was I decided not to take any chances being near the positive ions. An interesting sight filled the night. Electrical bolts lit up the house resembling a scene from the Boris Karloff movie ''Frankenstein'' when the scientist brought him to life. *Zzzzz.* Crackling electricity filled the air. *Fascinating.*

The roofer returned promptly November 1 and finished his job. The rains fell hard an hour later! (So traumatized was I by now that only two days are recorded in my diary between October 28 and November 11.)

Veteran's Day brought another healing crisis. But it was different from the others: severe sore throat, neck and shoulder pains, flu-like symptoms, weak, chills, sneezing, kidneys aching, feverish, multicolored stools. Why, it was like a *normal* healing crisis! Surprisedly I realized I'd had no symptoms of the disease for three weeks! Vasculitis — gone, arm pain — gone, cerebrals — gone, anaphylaxis — gone. The light was magic; I blessed Orie.

And I also phoned him with the stupendous news — he was delighted. Orie once more further enlightened me with some more news. ''The light balances positive and negative ions in the body thereby regenerating calcium, phosphorus, and magnesium, three essential minerals that are depleted and destroyed by the toxicity [especially by each reaction]. When the minerals come back'', Orie added, ''The body begins balancing itself. The intestinal flora will now regenerate on its own.'' He was right, for the vitamins and minerals I'd been taking up til now didn't feel as if they were assimilated. With the light I felt such tremendous body changes and instant pep that I was able to cut out most of them. In order to know what my body required, I began using the pendulum on a daily basis. In this way I discovered how little outside help I now needed. However, I still needed Orie. In fact, so impressed was I with Orie's knowledge that I invited him to speak at our HEAL meeting in January. ''Yup. I'll be there.'' A gift this man, a gift.

After the crisis, even greater changes continued on the light throughout November: the cellulite began disappearing on the back of my legs; the vaginal yeast disappeared; only my face turned red at AA meetings; my hair continued regenerating brown. Old joint pain resurrected, reminiscent of rheumatic fever at age 7, ending suddenly leaving the affected joints stronger; relived my back symptoms and fractured clavicle at age 19 which lasted about a week. Miraculously I felt ''something'' solid form in my spine where doctors had removed chunks of my fifth lumbar vertebrae years ago; my back felt fused, solid for the first time in my life!

Three days of cloudy, acidy urine accompanied all these changes along with a huge amount of energy. Mr. Bachechi predicted this, stating the body was throwing off heavy poisons — petrochemicals specifically. No symptoms for the past six weeks with the exception of the smoke inhalation reaction.

More curious than ever now about what was going on physically with me, I called on my expert — Orie. He said — ''The light has gotten to the intestinal flora. Presently, regeneration of it has begun. You will see faster and faster healing Elizabeth. You're on your way to health. It takes about 18 months for complete regeneration of the body. The central nervous system is the toughest to heal. It will be the last part to mend.'' Knowing I had neurotoxic poisoning, and remembering his earlier prediction that the light balances the body, his evaluation seemed correct. Yet somewhere inside me I knew recovery would happen sooner.

For healing of my heart began in November. The turbulent love-hate affair with Jean-Pierre reached its bitter end. The loneliness, the deep pervasive emptiness of this situation, forced me to re-evaluate my physical status. *If only I would trust better things would come my way, I could let him go.* Crying, frustrated, and anxious, I phoned Zena. ''Please help me, I'm grieving so. Staying with him was equal to letting him go. Had the time come to give up a man as a ''fix'' when I was ill, or was I being to hard on myself?'' Zena said the latter pointing out reality to me — ''You're sick, alone, isolated and terrified of the environment. Letting him go is cutting off your own nose right now.'' Unless, unless . . .

Yes, that was it — seek options! What was I well enough to do? Write. So I wrote to 8 men in the slick L.A. singles magazine, ''Intro.'' Take the risk, reach out. Risk being rejected with my disease. That's where it's at — risk and rejection, the double-edged sword. Why, I creatively even though up an ad for myself:

Wanted, single male, moderately sane. Blue Cross premiums
paid up. Preferably on the board of Prudential Health Insurance.

Brenda laughed uproariously when I shared my plot. We both had such severe physical limitations and high medical bills that the owner of the health insurance company seemed the only suitable mate!

An even greater idea entered my head. Start a support group for E.I. with the HEAL members I knew who wanted recovery. What an answer! I phoned five of them. Yes, love to. We'll be there. Tom had spoken to me several times in between our first meeting. His usual uplifting, enthusiastic self, he said he'd be glad to give me any help I needed. His offer softened my heart. Someone offering *me* assistance, and *with the disease himself*. Special person.

We set the date for the first meeting — November 22 — at my house. In order to accomplish this I had to strip my dining room bare so that the people wouldn't go into reactions from the accoutrements.

This action freed me to deal with Jean-Pierre. That night I dreamt of Jean-Pierre lying to me and dumping him from my life. Keeping him around, for any reason, was too much of a price to pay. As the holidays grew closer, my resentment toward him grew stronger as I remembered the previous seasons, especially the abuse Christmas of '81 when I was dying.

What abuse you say? No, I didn't mention this earlier because, in my initial writing, I tried to fudge a little on the truth, for Jean-Pierre looked so bad. But I can't leave it out, or you will feel a blank in my story.

Christmas of 81, Jean-Pierre did fly me to L.A. But, as soon as he dropped me at his house, he was leaving to spend the day with the-almost-ex-wife and children at her parents in Beverly Hills! We'd been arguing that morning in Berkeley about this. When he threatened to leave me there alone and dying if I didn't comply with his wishes I, desperately, acquiesced.

As Jean-Pierre walked out the door on me leaving me unable to cook, eat or barely survive alone, I screamed at him, "If you leave me now, we're finished." He left anyway. Through triple vision, I fell exhaustedly on his bed, phoned Zena, and raved about him to her. She couldn't believe what he'd done; she had no answers other than to listen to me. After I'd exhausted her sympathy (about 2 hours worth), I paced the streets slowly breathing in the clean, winter air. An attempt to attend an AA meeting was abortive. Everything went black before my eyes, as the cigarette smoke filtered into my body. Barely conscious, I fell out the door and just made it to Jean-Pierre's car to drive myself to his house, before complete exhaustion hit and I collapsed.

Jean-Pierre arrived at 7pm. I railed at him. He threatened to beat me up; I was defenseless. Knowing he meant it, I stopped, secretly telling myself, *one day I will be well and I will be gone — forever . . . .*

To dispose of this dreadful relationship, I had to forgive him in order to release myself. For the despair of my plight was upon me. Brenda left November 17 and Jean-Pierre departed for Palo Alto the next day, leaving me feeling deserted and abandoned by the world.

But the despair of that weekend was not wasted. The illness was mostly beyond my control - Jean-Pierre wasn't. After I decided to let him go, I realized my rage was at myself for my helplessness in the situation, for the cage my condition locked me into, and for the abuse I allowed him to foster on me. With this wisdom, I wrote a long list of all my resentments, both of him and me, followed by a list of amends to myself, beginning with "I forgive myself for I am isolated and very ill, and would have died without some intimate human warmth in my life," ending with, "I am awake now, less naive . . . believe my inner voice and trust it . . . won't allow a man to treat me this way again."

This decisive moment of incredible courage, gave me the stamina to cut the Gordian knot. And the success of the first E.I. meeting further strengthened my reserve. The program I outlined to heal our disease as I had done, was met with spectacular enthusiasm. Tom arrived shining like a Christmas tree. Hugs were shared all around. Touch. Precious touch. Tom really aided me a lot for he was already on the spiritual path. His presence brought healing joy to the meeting.

I liked him. Brilliant, marvelous humor, caring, cuddly, warmhearted, and full of ideas for recovery. A bright star in all this darkness. We became immediate friends. The others I began teaching muscle testing for nystatin and foods. The knowledge I shared with them, surprisingly, was unknown to any of them but me. Once more I was on my knees that night, thanking my Higher Power for giving me the physical vitality to initiate this desperately needed love system for our souls.

November 23 was Thanksgiving; November 24 was Jean-Pierre's 40th birthday: I refused vehemently to spend either one with him, screaming through the phone, ''I never want to see you again!'' I never did. — except for a brief period, six months later, during a life-threatening situation.

What a victory for my soul! I stood my ground and followed through despite several more phone calls from him. And it was the best Thanksgiving I ever lived. Free from Jean-Pierre, the pain of my children going to their fathers for the holiday, of my divorce, my crippled back, my alcoholism, and well on my way to freedom from candidiasis. Did I have a lot to be grateful for! At an AA meeting that day, a fellow AA invited me to her house for dinner. Anxiously, afraid only of cigarette smoke, I got up my courage and went. Inside the house was okay — outside was a very unhappy, 17 year old nephew of hers, with whom I chatted humorously. Mary was very kind to me. She mentioned filming my story for television before I left. Great! The world needs to be told this monstrous disease exists, and that there is hope.

Tom dropped by my house. We gabbed for hours. His grandfather invented a famous chocolate drink. He was an amateur inventor himself. Interesting person. I told him of my breakup with this long relationship. He listened compassionately, supporting my gutsy decision all the way. ''Why don't we go out together Tom, just as friends? You would help reduce a great deal of stress for me in re-entry, because you understand my dilemma.'' He loved the idea, for he knew the loneliness of the disease, and the inability to have any intimate relationship while in the acute throes of it. My heart lightened. For Tom, despite his lifelong suffering, had a wonderful attitude, with a keen sense of humor that made him a delightful companion.

Tom invited me to share Thanksgiving dinner with his family. ''No, thank you,'' I declined graciously. The stress of being in an unknown home, with people who have no comprehension of what I'm going through, was more than I could cope with right now. He understood, kissed me, and bid me *adieu*. Rain drenched the latter part of the holiday, so I went to see a movie, *Brainstorm*, and ate tons of popcorn. Very happy day!

So the fear of letting go of Jean-Pierre was unfounded. Releasing him brought multiple additions into my life all at once. And multiple fear, for re-entry is a long difficult process, especially in view of the fact that E.I. is akin to agoraphobia emotionally, the exception being that chemicals could *really* harm me seriously. Getting accustomed to after-shave, perfume and cigrarette smoke not placing you in life-threatening shock, takes the nerves of a gladiator and all the hanging on the apron strings of the Creator that is possible. Alone, up til now, I'd faced re-entry solo, except for the rare occasions in which Jean-Pierre would accompany me. For I tried the freeway alone. Too anxiety provoking, the fear being, I'd lose consciousness, someone would call the over-enthusiastic paramedics, and they'd kill me by, samaritanically, infusing dextrose and water into my veins, or worse yet, adrenalin with phenol.

That Thanksgiving weekend changed everything! I wasn't alone anymore. Yes, I had God, but we do live on the physical plane. The little network of five people brought me more than I dreamed. Friday morning, I had calls from two members, thanking me; Friday afternoon I saw ''Yentl'', identifying strongly with Streisand's struggle to survive as a very talented artist in the male-dominated movie industry; Friday evening, I continued adapting AA's big book to our disorder. Quite a challenge, since our reactions, before treatment, are beyond our control; Friday night I realized my life's work was in front of me.

A new me emerged that weekend: a new acceptance of my condition. Unapologetically, I told a very sympathetic shoe salesman I'd be measured in the street for an addition to the too-narrowlegged boots, because the glue in the shop was lethal to me. I didn't care what he thought.

That Saturday, Abe, the manager of the Music Center, who had candidiasis and myelofibrosis and whom I'd helped, had offered me free tickets to the shows anytime he had some. I took him up on his offer and phoned him, asking to see what he could do for Sunday. In the meantime, Tom phoned to invite me to the Beatles Annual Convention at the Bonaventure, in downtown L.A. I accepted, knowing he'd take me home if I couldn't ''tolerate'' the hotel. Super! For I'd realized by now that the others in our group were not life-threateningly ill as I was, and could assist me in re-entry. More comfort.

The Beatles outing was hilarious. Tom drove the nighttime freeway, which I wasn't ready to do. The gas heat at the hotel didn't bowl me over, so I was on my way. Together we faced the ''outsiders''. We told the attendants we couldn't be stamped with ink. ''Why?'' Tom blurted out ''allergy'', and I, ''toxicity''. Didn't matter. The strange looks were humorous. We enjoyed our Martian status because we shared it. We actually turned it around and made it a delight. Ironically, the ''normies'' had pink hair and blackened eyes. Who were the real weirdos?

We needed special permission from ''Mark'', a radio announcer and promoter of this production. No questions asked. He gave us permission slips to enter, just like grade school. Our oddity became lighthearted and comforting. After browsing through the memorabilia — mugs, records, buttons, tiny T-shirts — we ventured toward the huge auditorium screening Beatles films endlessly.

I was okay in there, but the true okayness came from not having to explain my situation to my companion. A no-anxiety evening — a true healer of the mind and body.

Presently, a band from Liverpool appeared to perform a medley. After singing, stomping and dancing with our hands, Tom asked me to dance with him up front by the stage among the teenagers going wild. A little afraid I'd collapse from the strain, I at first said no, then yes. Off we went to shake and sweat to "Hey Jude". *It was marvelous.* As the perspiration dripped down my black outfit, I thanked God for every drop. And for this evening. Around midnight, we left when people started lighting up cigarettes in the auditorium. Tom and I gabbed till 2am. What a night!

Thought I wouldn't be able to move the next day, but I could. Abe phoned with two tickets for the Joffrey that very day. Dazedly I called Jean, a group member, to join me. "Yes", she said — and I was ready to try driving the freeway downtown. Recalling turning gray, then suddenly being semi-conscious, I asked Jean if she could take over if I had to stop. "Sure." A great comfort. Off we went. I drove very slowly. Near Figueroa street, the Harbor-Santa Monica freeway interchange, I became very dizzy. But I made it.

The Ballet was lovely, until a woman sat down next to us with heavy perfume. Chills and faintness. Suddenly, I realized — I forgot to eat! So I really was okay, just needed food. What a relief. Panic was already setting in. But Jean was having trouble too. We left the theater grabbed some food and went to the car. "A Santa Ana condition exists today . . ." blared the radio announcer. Explained a lot. The drive home was easy. Total exhaustion hit when I arrived. A lot of chemical exposure the past two days. Wiped out til 11pm when a surge of energy suffused my being. At 2:30am, finally coming down from my high, I turned on the air-conditioner and fell into a deep sleep.

The aftermath of all this activity evoked a strong need to withdraw from people the subsequent days. Even positive stress is too much initially. Must be approached slowly, I told myself. Everything was overwhelming me. A natural reaction to intense long term isolation. *Why, I still had my sanity.* How, I don't know. Re-entry made me realize how much I'd been through. I sat down again and cried those paradoxical tears — a shocking realization that each day less and less isolation filled my life because I *was* better — tears of joy, knowing in my heart I was almost well. Otherwise, the weekend was a huge success on many levels. Most of all it bolstered my confidence about going out. Life was being returned to me.

The last two nights of November I couldn't sleep. Overstimulated. Overloaded. The second meeting of our group, some members balked at the format. I didn't have the energy for the hostility (chemical reaction) that bursts from people with this illness. Had I bitten off more than I could chew? The answer seemed yes. Overburdened with mourning the loss of Jean-Pierre, the roof anxiety, the sump pump repairs — all on my back. On top of this I kept urinating every 3 minutes in a reaction from a hamburger bun with ketchup — two no-no foods. The evidence pointed to attempting to return to normal living too fast. Time to back off rest and recuperate — again. In fact, so busy was I living in November, that I failed to understand that before the KIVA light I wouldn't have been able to cope with any of these events. The light had miraculous powers!

Foul smelling urine opened the third month on the light. More detox. Weak from overdoing it, I vowed to rest more. Tom called to invite me to a holistic, spiritual workshop the next day, but I felt too overstimulated to deal with it so I passed. The negative stress continued; the other owners ignored the pump situation. Another burden on my back, for it was my house that would flood when the rains came again, not theirs. Angrily, I hired a cheap plumber who, half-way through the job, told *me* to hire an electrician to hook up the electrical! I couldn't believe this guy! I raved at him. "Either finish it or get out. I won't pay you." He finished it. "It" finished me.

Between the outside stress and the inability to sleep til 3, 4, and 5am many nights, I felt myself rapidly going under emotionally. When I realized I'd paid for overkill physically setting myself back a bit, it dawned on me that returning to life would be a much longer process than I originally anticipated. *Remember this piece of wisdom Elizabeth. Remember it.* For I'd reached the "snapping" point once more. Popcorn was all I had to assuage my anxiety.

Orie told me the not sleeping was also the immune system kicking in. That eased my mind. *This too would pass.* Hopefully my sporadic sadness and tears at Jean-Pierre's departure would pass swiftly too. For as I decorated for the holidays, I missed him. Forgot the bad. Wished I could call him. But when I got this lonely, I remembered also that I didn't miss his chronic self-pity and negativity. *This too would pass.*

Strange but beautiful changes occurred in December: my hair became light reddish-blond — childhood's color. On the 2nd, along with chest discomfort, I began a transient tasting of cigarette tobacco. A phone conference with Orie enlightened me. "You're being rejuvenated back through childhood Elizabeth" he explained, "The cigarette taste is your lungs beginning to empty out all the nicotine and tar embedded in them from 20 years of smoking." And if that wasn't enough, my dreams took on a new, exciting turn. This excerpt is from my dream diary of December 3rd:

> *Suddenly, a voice tells me Amy is reborn — a beautiful baby is handed to me — free of allergies and all disease — a second chance. Head is very large. Inspect the whole baby, and it's reborn and perfectly healthy.*

Amy, as I came to know by keeping records, is me. Was the dream prophetic? We shall see.

December 10 brought two more miracles. I had a tree trimming party! Tom, that incredible person, celebrated with me and my girls. He brought presents for everyone — a book of his poems for me and skeleton keys wrapped in holiday colors for the girls to make a wish upon. We laughed, danced, ate, and sang. A merry night was had by all.

So merry in fact that I stayed up talking and laughing with Tom til 4am. Many hugs and kisses later we bid each other good day. Saturday I was so out of whack that I rapidly learned my limits. Between withdrawal from nystatin and grieving for Jean-Pierre, and Brenda's absence, my heart, mind and body were overloaded. Lack of sleep, despite the uplifting reason for it, quickly knocked me over physically. The loss of my only two human connections *without* the ailment whom brought other topics into my life was still devastating me. Much as I liked Tom, I didn't want to be around sickness anymore. The meeting I'd started was overwhelming me for my offer to help was greeted too needily by the others. Yes, compassion I had for them, but I also was re-entering life — it was simply too much for me. Why I was living as if I'd *not* been through all this! Paradoxically, I looked so well no one would believe I'd ever been sick at all. That's the rough part. Compassion begins at home — that was my lesson for the day.

For my big question was how and where do I meet normal people when I've been so seriously ill for so long and re-entering life? *It feels like I'm starting life all over again which boggles my mind.* The thought of a meeting the next Tuesday was more than I could bear. Too, too much — or I wouldn't be so upset.

Exhaustion, stormy and fire ridden dreams, and crying at my AA support group for my breakup with Jean-Pierre the following day, drove me to realize I was so overstressed I had to stop everything. The final straw came when Amy missed her bus to Westwood for her dyslexia teaching and she asked me to drive her — I burst into tears. Was that enough to prove I was overwhelmed? With that I promised myself that my goal for the month of December was to enjoy the life I'd missed since December of 1981.

Overload. Took me the rest of the week to settle down. During that period I had two astounding dreams. The first went:

> *Driving thru network of underground tunnels . . . Police are hiding in deep dark tunnels . . . I'm with someone(?) in a car . . . Policeman stops us searching for drug — finds none . . . Someone begins driving again . . . I'm in back seat measuring out a dose watching for police out car windows . . . We are stopped again and nystatin is confiscated . . . I don't care . . . I'll get more and continue my journey . . .*

My determination to heal despite obstacles was evidenced by this dream. But the other one took on an entirely different and hopeful note:

> *I'm very slim, dressed all in black— hat & veil, dress, nylons, and shoes, with a red carnation in my hair . . . Fashionable and Chic . . . It's Jen and Amy's day to be baptized or confirmed (or rewarded) in a church ceremony at St. Patrick's Catholic Church . . . We live in New York . . . Our life has changed completely . . . Presently, we're in a rented room number 74 . . . We roam the city waiting for our turn at the Cathedral . . . See two priests in white come out the side doors . . . There is beautiful singing inside . . . I ask when it will be childrens turn . . . Soon he says . . . I say let's dash off and change to pretty dresses for the event . . . Jen says no . . . Amy yes . . . We go jauntily to our apartment near the East or Hudson River . . . It's number 74 . . .*

Having studied a little bit about dream symbols, my curiosity piqued. Blue-green door — liberation. Number 74 adds up to eleven which is physical mastery. It appeared twice. I don't know what I will master but I feel it means whatever it is will transpire in eleven days — December 26. For many months I'd had a feeling candidiasis would disappear by Christmas. I pray it is true.

Thursday the 13th brought more withdrawal symptoms: head tightening, mental fogginess, paranoid thinking, slurred speech, numbness in left arm. Dr. Luc came to see me at home. Full of compassion. He mentioned he'd been studying our disease and was even more convinced the spleen was the main organ malfunctioning, causing the entire syndrome. An acupressure treatment cleared up the problem in five minutes. Nystatin had been discontinued five days earlier. Malathion was being sprayed near the Civic Center bringing enough to Santa Monica via the Santa Anas to affect me adversely. At the same time, I'd begun "Nature's Sunshine" taheebo, which was much stronger than the brand I'd been using. This combination reminded me once more how vulnerable my body still was physically. While going off nystatin, I'd also added black walnut herb, a natural antifungal, to my daily comfrey and licorice root. I wasn't taking any chances this time going off nystatin.

Heavy fog permeates Santa Monica throughout the rainy season (November to May) usually resurrecting the brain symptoms in me. Wondrously, the suicidal cerebrals had disappeared completely! Agitation and some eye irritation were the only symptoms bothering me — minor compared to olden days. A negative-ion machine plus air conditioning at night alleviated my discomfort totally, along with taking three calcium tablets, and an immunplex as a "sleeping pill." This discovery ended my sleepless nights.

Fruit came back into my life on a limited basis during December. A persimmon, a tangerine — I suckled each bite, each drop of juice as if I'd been handed the nectar of heaven.

The grieving for Jean-Pierre hit me harder and harder as the holidays progressed. My diary wept:

that one right now. Reminding myself that I was not alone —
Zena, Brenda, children, Tom and God. No longer would I be
attracted to ''the package'' — the gilt, but the inner essence of
the man. At last, I knew the difference. My ex-husband and Jean-
Pierre were all show!!

I couldn't sleep from the grief, so I sat and watched ''The Song of
Bernadette'' til 3am. She was a Catholic saint. I'm not, but I have suffered
beyond belief and not lost faith. A lesson was learned from her life. *Accept
my suffering as a gift from God.* In the early morning hours I thanked my
Lord on bended knee and surrendered my health to my Creator to do with it
what *He* willed.

My diary continues the next morning:

My bleeding heart days seem to be over. A dream last night
showered me with tons of manna from heaven — I walked
through a giant bakery of any and all kinds of bread. I was
handed a rod to hold on to. The baker offered me any bread I
desired (in real life I couldn't touch bread). I take the loaves. I go
to a subway. The conductor holds a rod between me and himself.
All of a sudden I'm moving rapidly in the room. Then a door
opens and we zoom along plain corridors. I'm on my way home.

My dream book said the rod is discipline earned through suffering. The
baker was God. Through this type of dream I gratefully received nourishment (the manna) I wasn't getting on planet earth.

Surprisingly that very same day, my girls remained with me for the
weekend (Dad cancelled last minute). What a boost to me who dreaded
being alone right then! We saw two movies, one of them, the memborable
''The Keep'', a metaphysical horror story set in the Tyrolean Alps during the
Nazi occupation. Later on that evening I sat with Jen in her bed, listening to
her tell me she didn't deserve good things. I don't know if that's just being a
teenager or something I should be concerned about. Don't know much, but
willing to learn. For only by being so ill had I learned to love myself. Now, I
was well enough to share this knowledge with her and teach her how to
believe that she did deserve good things. Grateful, just plain grateful.

Even further blessings were bestowed upon me. The journal continues:
December 28, 1983 — a gift was given to me tonight. A man
called Tom. As the scar of pain began ripping apart in my gut, as I
cried to Zena, about using the man as a fix, avoiding the pain, the
doorbell rang. I grabbed him and threw his arms around me
asking him to hug me. He did and I spewed forth my pain and
agony — the mental madness that descends upon me from the
corridors of the brain . . . the abuse . . . the old abuse by my
father . . . He sat with me as I bulged my insides, ready to rupture
with agony. He held my hand as I blurted out ''Don't come on to
me, don't come on to me — I'll kill you''. The dam burst, the tears
flooded. He continued to hold my hand — an ''I care'' gesture.

Shortly thereafter the pain subsided and I felt fine. Believe it or not, we went out for a delightful evening. Off to Westwood in my car with the ''Iron pig'' (the filter) as my girls called it. ''Terms of Endearment'' was the agenda. We laughed our heads off, while sniffing the seats next to us for after-shave and perfume.

Somewhere, in the midst of the movie, I glanced at Tom and felt a pang of softness, nurturing, a flick of feeling I'd call love, but I pulled away from it as it was premature in my delicate condition. Back home, I played with Tarot cards. Although he said he enjoyed it, he looked anxious. Tom's insides were unmasked before my very eyes. He was shaken. Confusion and disillusionment are his present friends, acceptance his greatest virtue, rebirth his future. Great fun. After many hugs and a half-hour goodbye we parted for the night.

December 21 brought peace into my life. The big secret the man was covering up was my fear of abandonment during this illness. The previous night with Tom began my liberation from my deepest form of self-destruct — falling in love with highly disturbed men. Peaceful, peaceful day. Happiest Christmas season in my whole life. Shopped for last minute presents — one for Tom too. Though totally exhausted, I wrapped all the presents myself that night. Three days before Christmas. *I can't believe it!*

A dream during the night showed me convalescing in a hospital. Next a single red rose appeared in a basket in a mountain pass, through which water flowed peacefully. All symbols of healing. The war was over. I would be free of this illness! Just didn't know when.

The month became funnier and funnier. I attended a male, gay, AA meeting to walk through the pain of my male obsession. Since they were obsessed with males too, they were very loving and supportive. Met a sexy fellow named Mark — too bad he was gay. Compassion flowed from them for AIDS had stricken their community severly and they understood my sister-disease as the slow, torturous death it was. Why, all my needs were met here! *And no smoking too.*

The pain appeared again December 23. Cried. Went to church and broke down crying over my mother's death four years earlier. Needing more support, I attended an OA (Overeaters Anonymous) meeting where the support and warmth I needed were supplied to stop me from binging on forbidden foods, especially peanuts and sugar during my mourning period.

Christmas Day — the most wonderful one of my life! Free of destructive male relationships, the ghost of my marriage, the feelings of abandonment when the girls leave for the holidays with their father, and negative people. So near to well from my illness, I can taste it!

Amy returned from the vacation with her Dad an absolute mess emotionally, her huge brown eyes looking broken hearted. Seems no one filled her stocking with anything at her Dad's but styrofoam; I'd only placed two small gifts in hers. No candy or toys! She was sad and miserable. I comforted her telling her we'd fill up the stocking tomorrow. She felt a little better. As I tucked her young body in bed I hugged her again and again. Talked some more. Powerless to change things that night, I comforted her pain. She finally fell asleep to the sound of the TV set running incomprehensibly in front of her.

The biggest surprise of the night was Tom. He gave me a book of poems written by him about how he felt surviving this illness. A secret piece of himself. A dedication in the front wished me well. ''No more dragons to slay,'' and thanked me for my inspiration and love. He then declared me a miracle walking. Deeply touched, I hugged him to pieces. Then he gave me a membership in the ''Hug Club'' — I liked that.

Jen was another surprise. I've never seen her so animated. She flipped when she saw the grey *Le Sport Sac* bag — and rollerskates with blue wheels . . . and a grey wallet. ''Mom, this is the first Christmas I got everything I wanted.'' Glad to see her so happy.

And last but not least, an incident on Christmas Eve proved a stiff test of my resolution not to use sex to avoid my feelings.

That morning after attending an OA meeting I went home to prepare myself for a few last minute errands before the stores closed. But first I wanted to pick up the mail. I opened the patio door — and shock of all shocks — there stood Jean-Pierre putting presents in my mailbox. I began to shake. *Oh no, please don't let me give in Lord.* He said he had a Christmas present for me. Stiffly, I told him I didn't want it as strong feelings of sexual desire cascaded throughout my body and memories of tenderer times flooded my brain.

Jean-Pierre said ''Take it'' softly. I ignored him. ''Let me hug you for Christmas.'' I did, stone cold.

''You look lovely — so healthy.''

''Thank you.''

''Where are the girls?''

''At their Dad's for the holiday.''

''You're alone?'', he said sadly.

''Yes,'' as tears began to swell in my eyes. ''Only alone right now — not for the holiday,'' I blurted cheerily letting him know through silence I was seeing someone.

That old seductive devil of compassion and holding me stood right in front of me. Yes, I needed them. I'd nearly succumbed to these emotions, getting ready to drag Jean-Pierre upstairs to my bed, when he said, ''I'm late to pick up my children.'' *That did it!* All the memories of Christmases past flooded me; I became steel. All the pain puked out at once.

I gave the gift back. He placed it inside my door. Icily I uttered ''Goodbye. You don't know how to let go.'' His eyes filled with tears. *Manipulation, Elizabeth, rang loudly in my head, those tears are not for you, or us, but for him drowning in his own self-pity.* I wanted to be rid of him. He left, dejectedly.

Back inside the house I fought back the sickening pain in my gut. I tried to concentrate on my tasks but my head reeled. I broke down pouring years of sadness from my insides. I called Zena. She was there for me. I needed her. "It feels as if satan himself came to the door. This was a test of my surrender to God of love relationships. Of trust."

"I won, I made it, I steeled myself to him," I wept my pain to her. "It worked. I made it — I didn't drink, use sex, stuff food, or bury myself in work. With of course, a great deal of help from my Higher Power. A wonderful miracle!" Zena agreed.

Afterwards I attended Christmas Eve Mass at St. Monica's Church. I chatted animatedly with an elderly lady next to me. The church was resplendent with poinsettias gracing the pure white altar while candled douglas firs hugged her sides. The sight was so wondrous I cried on and off throughout the Mass. *Jesus came to save us from our sins — that was the miracle of his birth.* Was this the church I was going into in the dream ten days ago? The colors I wore were the same — red sweater and black corduroy slacks. Then I noticed stained glass windows similar to my dream the night before. Was this what all these dreams were leading to?

At home once again I phoned my friends — my sister Dee in New York, Judy Smith in Las Vegas, and Joelynn in Palos Verdes. Joelynn tried to make my friendship with Tom into a love affair. "No," I protested, "We're just friends, that's all." Then Tom arrived and we went to midnight Mass. The sight was like a subway at rush hour — one barely could see the magnificent altar for the crowds standing in the aisles.

When the assembly disassembled we strode to the altar to pay homage to our Lord and Master. Tom, being Jewish and having a new experience, was deeply moved by the whole event. I sat down to pray. My shoulders turned to lead. So did Tom's. We didn't know what was happening, but experienced a deep peace flooding us.

And so it happened. My prophetic dream saying I'd be liberated from "something" to do with physical mastery in eleven days came to pass. On December 26, at 5:30am, I sleepily recorded the following:

I saw the healing of compulsion. A kaleidoscope appeared swirling endlessly pulling me with it (in spirit form) A Voice from the right side said, "This is how a person is healed. Healing is mentioned over and over again. (I went to bed in agony over sexual cravings and prayed for help.) Many multicolored wheels spinning with my spirit swirled among them, as if I were being taken apart and reassembled. The seven wheels were red, green, yellow, and blue in the center. As the healing took place, I felt extraordinarily peaceful and soothed. Compulsion (sex?) disappeared. Somewhere a hand was touching my head during the healing.

Can't remember the rest. Too incredible for words.

Recordings in my diary of December 28th further depicts my shocked reaction:

A few days are missing since my last entry for another incredible event has transpired, taking me several days to digest. On the morn of the 26th of December, just as my dream of the 15th revealed, I was liberated from something — I say that because I don't know the Creator's mind and refuse to guess at this point what mystical event has occurred. You see, I was suffering so deeply from my sexual compulsion that I rolled to and fro in bed, begging God to help me as the power of the compulsion paralleled, if not exceeded, my alcoholic obsession. So I prayed and eventually slept.

About 5am, I awakened from a dream so powerful, I actually felt the events in my body. In the dream I actually saw *how* God heals. Yes, I *saw* the healing of an abstract word such as compulsion. (I've become vague because I was so dazed when I bolted awake.) I woke up sweating and shook. This dream was followed by one of me as a nurse caring for a priest whose heart was seriously wounded, so I placed him in ICU. In the center of the floor was a huge box-shaped narcotics closet to which I'd been given the key. I opened the lock. Inside was an unfinished interior with a dirt floor and cases of narcotics in wooden crates. Most of the pills were yellow and orange. To me, this dream was about healing my heart underneath my compulsion, but only a part of it was revealed. The key opened the door to my attitude of sex as dirty and narcotizing myself not to feel my sex drive. But the whys and hows were not revealed.

Although it took me several days to calm down to record this writing, I believed I'd been healed very deeply physically. And mentally, for I wrote on the same night:

Tom, dear Tom, the hell we've both been through and the heaven we are about to receive. When we met in September, did we know we'd become such good friends? I think not. Of all the crowd surrounding me that 20th day of September, you were a special presence. A warmth flowed from you. Perhaps — what do I mean *perhaps* — God put us together. You are very special to me and your poems were a gift of yourself. I ''heard'' you and decided to let it be. We shall see what happens.

Tom was a very, *very* special man.

THE FINALE OF THE ILLNESS

The week after the healing dream was filled with miracles. Exposed to glue, tar, cigarette smoke, and perfume. No reaction! My body continued to pass odd material — gray-green stools. Then a strange occurrence transpired. My legs pounded, then my thighs, leading to my head which felt as if something were rotating clockwise inside of it followed by tightness at the base of my skull and teeth. This was rapidly succeeded by flu symptoms, *plain old flu* — sore throat, aching shoulders, tiredness and stuffed head. Nothing so ordinary had taken place in a very long time! Colonics produced huge amounts of brown mucusy chunks. When I called Orie with all this info, he deciphered that the brain symptoms were oxygen being released to starved cells while the flu symptoms were indicative of how cleansed my body was. When I told him about the changes in Amy's health — anaphylaxis to horse and animal dander disappeared, severe tree and weed allergies greatly diminished, only one throat infection since September (she usually had infections two or more weeks out of every month), large amounts of old penicillin passed in stools, and yellow-white material was released from her ears (old ear infections) — Orie was not the least bit surprised. In fact, he laughed heartily, reiterating, ''I told you the light detoxes everyone nearby. Now do you believe me?'' ''Yes,'' I stuttered ''Yes.'' What more could I say?

New Year's Eve came. Chest and shoulders inflamed (old bronchitis symptoms?), sore throat, blood in left nostril. Recollected old nosebleeds from rheumatic fever — signs of rapid healing as these symptoms were from childhood and teens — I was that far back in rejuvenation. But nothing could stop me now from enjoying life. Tom had invited me to a wedding at midnight; I was determined to go.

He brought me one red rose — a gift of love. The party went well. I lasted two hours amidst candles and exterior cigarette smoke. Did fine. A handsome man flirted with me outrageously. He asked me out. "I can't . . ." I stammered flustered . . . *Not yet, you don't know the truth, I'm not ready.* I bolted from him and stood next to Tom trembling, as the happy couple cut their wedding cake. Right near the end of the ceremony, I freaked. Felt myself bursting into tears. Grabbed Tom's hand, told him. He hugged me tightly and held me through the shaking. Outside, I felt better. This was a great night for me, for so certain was I that I was completely well that I ate cake, bagels, and regular food at the reception.

We left, driving the side streets, avoiding the anxiety of holiday traffic and car fumes, and went home. The girls were rollerskating in the street at 1:30am. The house looked like a confetti parade. As a matter of fact, the rainbow colors improved the look of the wornout carpeting.

New Year's always resurrected feelings about my ex-husband — anger — not love. I shared these with Tom. The urge to vomit came as I burst into tears. Tom hugged and caressed me for a long time. Unexpectedly, I felt a funny feeling in my heart or stomach; I know not which. I asked him to kiss me — he did — passionately. I liked it and was turned on, but stopped him.

No. Vulnerable. Too vulnerable. Don't start a love affair in that state. Tom respected my wishes. And held me, and held me, and held me as I burst into tears again. A wonderful human being.

Happy New Year to me! Zena was the first one filled with my Eve's tale when I woke up at lunchtime. Tom came by and took me to a party in Venice — there was none. Starved, we dined at the "Golden Arch." An easy day. We walked on Venice Beach, laughing and sharing past experiences. At his sister's in Venice, I phoned the girls. "Come home Mom," Amy said, missing me. I did. Tom looked awkward. He asked if he should leave. "Come on in and say hi." "Hi" lasted 4½ hours. The girls talked and talked to him, especially Amy. The evening was a treat — comforting.

As I summed up the holiday I was overjoyed. I didn't have a negative reaction to anything — that in itself was amazing. Plus I'd eaten cake.

Well, I didn't get away with it. Depression hit Monday night. By Tuesday I was in a full scale sugar reaction — spooked, spaced, crazy thinking. Sugar still *verboten*. A colonic released large amounts of brown mucus from my system. So I'd overdone it again *but I sure enjoyed it.*

You'd think by now I'd remember that when a "healing" occurs, the physical follows. Since I'd forgotten, my body reminded me. January proved very rocky. Fatigue began day in and day out. Lung pain started on the right side. Head hot and burning. Sore throat. Slept 10 to 12 hours per day. Aching in back of lungs, sweats, faintness. Walked. Almost passed out. Orie just happened to call in the midst of all this. "Body is cleaning out nicotine and alcohol." Colonics produced large amount of brown mucus with pieces of cigarettes (I used to eat butts as a child!)

Lots of old "alcoholic thinking" returned. Resentful, hypersensitive, angry but, able to laugh. *That was a switch.* Had to mean I was near the end of the line. The toughest part of this phase was being awake til 3, 4 and 5 in the morning again. And so it went, up all night — sleep all day. During this massive healing many old emotions which I'd held in, being so stoic, were pushed to the surface. The pain was so great I was forced to cry, rant, or pound it out on my pillow and floor. The release was powerful, further relaxing my body, and aiding my progress. The emotional agony was so strong I felt as if something were being ripped from every cell of my body. Probably true.

Sex cravings racked my body again. At the same time, I withdrew from Tom, sensing *his* neediness, not wanting to be drained by it. A winner in a bad place. But my sexual urges were part of my physical healing — for they were exaggerated beyond belief. Was I in a bind — fighting off my feelings toward Tom, while no outlet for the cravings save auto-eroticism. *An answer will come. Needed fun, pleasure to get through this.* No choice here. Due to my immune dysfunction, casual sex was more than a compromise — it could be my death warrant.

So back I went to the movies and simple childhood joys, like playing games with the girls and getting into their world more. That was the message of a magical fruit tree that appeared in a dream! Revert to childish pleasures to get through this.

Writing also helped, for through seeing where I was in a concrete form usually brought answers. Children don't have sex and I felt like a young child right now. I knew loving sex would be restored to me one day through choice not disease-induced physical cravings. A sense of humor was an absolute must too.

And one more thing. That day I read *Time* magazine's coverage of Pope John Paul II's forgiveness of his would-be assassin. The story was beautifully written by a very sensitive reporter trying to understand the true meaning of this act in a universal manner. My heart was touched by the article as a gush of tears sprung from my deeply scarred soul. Forgiveness — it brings freedom to the person forgiving. In my desperate hours I prayed to learn to forgive more thoroughly in order that I might be completely healed.

Weeks have passed since I wrote the previous chapter, the reason being I've been too busy writing books and enjoying life. However, I'll fill you in on what transpired between January and August 84 as I close this chapter.

A final massive healing crisis followed ''the healing dream'' in January. After that my energy was huge, but my psyche was scarred. Slowly, very slowly I began, truly this time, re-entering the world. *And nothing happened.* Flicks of loss hit me from time to time regarding Jean-Pierre but I didn't call him.

But the most interesting phenomenon to date was the apparent emotional healing that followed the detoxification with the KIVA lights.

During acute symptoms of cleansing — exhaustion, depression reliving your old symptoms — a simultaneous emotional regurgitation occurs. Every negative incident in your life reappears in no specific order. The longer you use the light, the deeper the emotional cleansing delves. I found myself re-experiencing events I'd suppressed or forgotten. But every event we've ever lived is stored somewhere in the body, which I suspect is the brain and the pathways of the nervous system. Therefore as your body heals, so do the emotions — spontaneously. I found this fact fascinating and wonderful! (New users of the light should be aware that this happens so they don't think they are going backwards.)

If the emotional or physical cleansing becomes too debilitating, I suggest you turn off the light, using it only to treat your food and water til it passes. Initially I found the light could be used for only an hour the first three days. And I'd been cleaning out for *two years* previously! Caution must be exercised however not to try to recover too rapidly. The symptoms will leave you virtually non-functioning.

Whatever this mysterious light did physically in my body I'm not exactly sure. I am sure however that the healing that took place, evidenced by migrating feelings of warmth or soreness to the damaged part, released simultaneously, old emotional traumas. To me this was nothing short of miraculous, for it went beyond psychiatry — the spirit healed. In my case that brought about a true and permanent healing.

Today I'm convinced, were I to reproduce the events that led to my breakdown — ignoring physical limits, over-achieving, returning to a toxic diet, or alcohol or toxic thinking, and severe stress — I could resurrect the entire disease. The lesson for me was to change to a loving attitude toward myself. With that, I believe, one will not re-experience the same sickness. Let me give an example here.

All was going extremely well for me after January: gradually going off nystatin whose positive side effect was a twenty-pound weight loss; totally discontinuing Pau D'arco; Tom joyfully assisting me to re-enter life; letting go of Jean-Pierre emotionally; being able to eat fruit and restaurant food without ill effect; being able to allow my children's friends in the house with shampoo and hair conditioner on their person; re-joining AA for moral support; and being able to dance, ride my bike, rollerskate and play without collapsing. Life seemed magical. Of course there were everyday crises, and the expected overdoing it, then withdrawing — I didn't become perfect — just human. Each setback was a lesson. Try one new food at a time, go off nystatin one tiny dose at a time while taking the chemex and kantita to reduce withdrawal. Insidiously the KIVA light continued its very subtle healing. After the first 90 days, the changes are virtually unnoticeable; what is noticeable is that you become aware *nothing is happening* when exposed to perfume, after shave etc.

So what went wrong on April 22, Easter Sunday, when I visited my old friend Theresa's house with Jen for dinner? The night before I'd attended a

Pascal Mass in which 1,000 candles were lit while the congregation held hands singing the "Our Father." If that didn't indicate I was well, nothing did! Confidently I entered Theresa's home Easter morn noticing the brand-new carpeting. *I'll be allright.* The gas cooking I entirely forgot. By the end of dinner, my head pounded and I felt severely nauseated. *It will subside,* I reassured myself.

The next morning, there, right across from my house's second story bedroom window, were roofers preparing to re-tile my neighbor's single-story house. Fear struck, then a calm voice saying, *ignore them, you'll be all right.*

That wasn't the truth. Anaphylaxis followed. This episode was reminiscent of the pesticide poisoning the previous September in its seriousness. *What would I do without Jean-Pierre?* The roof provided a new horror: for the first time in my illness, evacuation of my home would be necessary to my survival.

I crawled to Dr. Luc, where so blasted was I by the formaldehyde emanating from the cans of black substance the roofers used, that I collapsed in his office, turning yellow. Luc was extremely concerned "Get out Elizabeth, your energy is so low, one more exposure will be it — we'll lose you."

When Luc was this concerned, he verified my feeling that death awaited me there. Totally panic stricken, and with a rapidly fogging brain, my mind raced over whom I could move in with. Who knew my story? Who would help and comfort me? Jean-Pierre was the only logical answer.

You must realize by now the desperation of my plight to call him. Life and death forced me to forget, for the time being, the ugly words that had flown between us. At the same time, despair and confusion set in — *Why, Lord, why?* I believed this was over for me. *Why?* The answers would come.

Jean-Pierre wholeheartedly agreed to let me stay. He was also involved with a new woman which he neglected to tell me, but I discovered, as I smelled perfume on the "female" side of his bed. Half-dead, I had to strip the toxic sheets, replacing them with my own cotton ones. Jean-Pierre arrived at 9:30pm. Automatically, I cried, he held me, we went to bed. Halfway through lovemaking, I whispered, "I love you" in his ear. His entire being went limp. Something was very wrong.

The next morning I discovered two terrible facts: he was sexually *and emotionally* involved with a new woman; he hated me and wanted revenge. What a trap! What possible lesson could be in this, when physically, I was close to death. How much more negative stress could enter my life without me cracking or dying?

A *new* inner voice saved me during this period, for I became painfully aware that Jean-Pierre was highly emotionally disturbed, and that only a power greater than myself could get me through this one.

For the roof took weeks while the torture Jean-Pierre had in store for me vascillated between warmth and sadism. While I lay helplessly dying on his bed, he went about his job, his girlfriend, and his courses as if I didn't exist. Whenever he did appear at the house, he'd scream hysterically at me how I was a bitch who'd ruined his life, his job, and anything else he could think of. As sick as I was, I could see Jean-Pierre was certifiable.

Yet, the time at Jean-Pierre's was not wasted, for another giant healing came my way. April 28, 1984 is probably a day I will not forget for the rest of my life. The tension between Jean-Pierre and I reached explosion point rapidly. For he was going out with his new girlfriend that night (two days after I'd arrived there), and obviously going to have sex with her. *I went insane.* How could he do this *and* come home to me, full of her perfume and bodily exudates, with me here who wants his body, but not him! Me, who had barged in on him in a life and death situation out of nowhere, after five months of an ended love affair.

For three days, my body ached with lust for him, while my body was being strafed with allergic shock, severe chemical depression, and crying. Obsessively, I went over in my mind many ways to seduce him to make love to me. Who cared that he had a new girlfriend — that made it all the more imperative I get what I wanted. Early on, he'd told me, *after the brief fling,* he wouldn't touch me, that he could only handle one woman at a time, or lose his sanity: I believed him.

But my ''need'' kept torturing me. *If I could just have my sexual needs met — just one episode — I'd go into the sunset and say goodbye.* In other words, I wanted to use him and he wouldn't let me. I was enraged.

Friday evening, he yelled and yelled at me about how awfully *I* had treated him, (forgetting totally all his self-centered, cruel behavior). A part of me thought he was nuts, while somwhere inside me I knew there was a smidgen of truth in what he said.

A new softness came over me which I'd lost surviving my alcoholic father. In that moment I saw the pain in Jean-Pierre's heart — that he loved me and lost me because he wasn't enough for me, and I'd hurt him badly by pointing out his shortcomings so brutally to him. (Believe me, I did not forget for one minute his abusive behavior towards me.) I guess at this juncture, forgiving Jean-Pierre began. For he was obviously tormented by his own desires for me (he'd made sexual advances to me then pulled away just as abruptly over the past few days), wanting to shuck the life he'd been building since I threw him out last November, and fall at my feet again. How that poor soul loved me! But my compulsion was stronger than his truth. Although we parted for separate outings for the night, the sexual issue wasn't resolved.

My ''date'' was my spiritual teacher, an American-born kahuna (a Hawaiian priest), who held meditation and spiritual teaching services every Friday night. Drained of every ounce of energy in my body, all I could do was cry. Tom was present, and held and hugged me. I asked Dr. King why my immune disease had disappeared then reappeared suddenly on Easter Sunday. He replied compassionately, ''Your emotional body needs more healing. It is weakened. Then the physical will heal. Take very good care of yourself and your body will heal." (The full impetus of this explanation would not hit me til a later date.) The kahuna then said, "I will transfer energy to you as yours is very low." He told me, "Say to yourself *I'll be well,* for God has chosen you for something special. Visualize your body well, travelling, enjoying life." To which I blurted through tears, "God loves me, God loves me!" I complained bitterly to him about being stuck with Jean.-Pierre "Ask God to show you the perfect place where you can heal." Suddenly, I felt alive, free of sickness, and ready for the Golden Arch.

Tom and I chugged there by car, stuffing ourselves with fries and burgers. Realizing I was still totally drained, I bid my friend good night and went back to Jean-Pierre's house.

I couldn't sleep. As the clock ticked away to 1, then 2, I quietly seethed with jealousy, seeing "them" in my mind's eye making love. My stomach was in endless knots. *God please help me.* The torture of my sexual compulsion kept shattering my brain — I'll surely snap if this continues.

When finally he arrived at 2am, the woman's perfume scent on him hit my nose; chest pain began on top of my severe restlessness and constant urinating. *God, I can't take this.* Angrily, I jumped out of bed to urinate. Upon my return, he touched my shoulder. I seethed with resentment. Again, I bolted from the bed, dragging all the covers with me, except for one flimsy sheet, which I left hanging off him. *Just because I was sick didn't mean I would stand for emotional abuse. No way!* I stumbled down the stairs in my rage, and plunked myself on his couch, twenty feet from the gas stove that would affect me. Jean-Pierre came down to talk to me, but I waved him away, yelling the perfume on his body was giving me chest pain.

I lay there all night seething. On and off I slept, but not peacefully. My mind raced obsessively — *she's not getting any if I can't.* (Negative *obsessive thinking is a result* of acute poisoning, and is *magnified* by negative social stress, which is what was happening here.) My jealousy was rampant. All I could think of was — I must move out of here. Yes, I was in the deadly position of having nowhere to go; yes, Jean-Pierre had opened his home to me — that was all. The pain in my gut became worse and worse. *God help me,* I cried again and again, *help me* — my obsession was killing me.

Saturday morning I arose and angrily began packing to leave with nowhere to go. My rage could no longer contain itself; I blasted Jean-Pierre for how he'd treated me in the past three days; he denied his lousy behavior.

Suddenly, I softened and laughed. "Jean-Pierre, you're guilty even if you don't do anything." He replied sheepishly, "That's true. I didn't have sex last night." Still, he seemed oblivious to his gauche treatment of me. I decided to let it go — the man was walled in by his defenses, and blocked off from his own behavior. We both laughed and called a truce . . . .

Later that afternoon, we were resting in his bed together; Jean-Pierre was asleep. I still wanted to seduce him. The phone rang and awakened him. So I decided to tell him my plan. "Jean-Pierre, please come here, I want to tell you something." Through tears, I said how I cared for him, wanted him, and finally would like to make love with him before we parted permanently. He said through smiles my idea lacked credibility. We both laughed. "No," he said, as if to a spoiled child wanting her candy, "For me, it will be a beginning again." It was then I knew and felt how deeply he still loved me; for me, it was only sexual desire that was left: I had to release him. I shook my head no, then hugged him tightly, soaking his jogging jacket in my sad, sad tears. In that moment, forgiving Jean-Pierre progressed.

We hugged and hugged. I told him how I'd loved him for staying with me when I was so ill, for loving me through so many tough times, for visiting me in Berkeley and helping to keep me alive. We hugged again. I told him I was sorry for any hurt I'd given to him. Could he forgive me? Yes, he said softly. Yes, he'd hurt me too, but we'd already been through that one far too many times without resolving anything.

Something changed between us in that moment. I saw him in a new light — not the big strong man he pretended to be, but as the flawed person he was. And I loved him freely in that instant. He seemed to drink up the caring.

The tension dissolved, I decided to fix us a simple dinner on my portable electric burners (Yes, I was pushing myself, but loving feelings seem to add some extra juice to the body). Lovingly, I prepared chicken breasts and steamed vegetables. Jean-Pierre joined me. Side by side, we helped one another prepare the meal. Then we agreed to forgive one another, have no sex, and hugs only. Laughter re-entered our lives as I hugged him every chance I got.

Nothing could have prepared me for what then transpired. We sat down to dinner whilst listening to Gilberto sing his dreamy, Portuguese love songs on the stereo. As I was about to pick up my fork, a corridor of my life from ages 4 to the present, in the form of a film strip, flashed before my eyes. I saw every man who'd ever been in my life go past my vision in lightning timing. My attitude towards all of them was changed for the better within seconds. I saw clearly, how it *was,* not how *I* saw it as a child. Simultaneously, I felt an invisible blow to my solar plexus that bolted me backwards in my chair. Grief poured down my face as I realized God had healed me in that instant, of all the scars in this area, which had set me on self-destruct at age four, after I'd been sexually molested by a stranger in Central Park. God had freed me of my past in one fell swoop.

Jean-Pierre looked at me puzzled. Amazingly, he looked almost like a different person to me. I saw a man so madly in love with me, he couldn't see straight; I also saw a person who had tried and failed with me, yet still loved me. I said these things to him. He leaned his chair against the wall weakly, nodding his head yes. I felt crappy for the way I had attacked him — so harshly and cruelly verbally. If I ever felt that incompatible with a man again, I would let him go, not repeat this behavior. A gigantic lesson. For both our psyches were severely lacerated from our cruel interchanges and put-downs. The more loving approach would be to let go with love. This is what I was now attempting to do.

Again, I told Jean-Pierre I was sorry from the bottom of my heart for any pain I had caused him. I let him know that I now knew he had given me his best, and that I was unable to see this due to my own emotional scars.

The impact of this experience on me was mind-boggling. I was grieving so heavily, I couldn't eat. *God had forgiven me, for I'd truly forgiven Jean-Pierre.* Thunder-struck, I sat there crying like a baby. Jean-Pierre asked what was wrong. I shared with him that "something" had been healed in me instantaneously. "Your trouble with men?" Yes. Again, Jean-Pierre appeared in a totally new light to me: I saw him only as an ordinary, fallible human being. Peace was made — for that night.

The peace didn't last. For Jean-Pierre, verbally, threw me out into the street the following Thursday of my incarceration; I fled voluntarily. Nowhere to go. I holed up at Brenda's apartment where a gas leak from her stove came close to ending my story. A day and a half was all I lasted at Brenda's, as the gas fumes sent me into suicidal depressions, and my body became waxen as I began to eventually lose consciousness. Fleeing her house at midnight, in order to stay alive (she'd gone out for the evening), I stopped first at my house. Within 15 minutes, my arms and upper torso had no feeling. My house was still toxic. Jean-Pierre's keys still in hand, half-conscious, knowing it was back to his house or die, somehow sufficient strength came to get me into my car, and drive back to his house where I literally fell in the door and collapsed on his couch. (He'd phoned my house frantically, in between my departure and rearrival, over and over, earlier the same day telling my children to tell me to come back.) Only through a miracle did I live through that night.

My diary, written several days later, details this other miraculous event:

> The stress of not knowing where Jean-Pierre was or if he'd come in to sleep with his girlfriend in front of me, prevented me from sleeping. I tossed and turned on his couch till 2am, then crawled up to his bedroom, not caring anymore if he came in or not. Dealing with the emotional pain of seeing Jean-Pierre with someone else (even though we were over), on top of my desperate situation, was enough to shatter my sanity. Over and over, I begged God first to help me, then to take me.
>
> Dozed off about 3am. I had a spectacular dream. It's very vague in my mind, but also very clear that it really happened. *I saw a mass of energy being sent from the Hawaiian islands. Hundreds of souls appeared above the mass, sending me healing energies. My body was bombarded by a solid, huge mass of pure energy coming down from the sky. Simultaneously, two bolts of energy joined forces from below [the mass] and united in a great bond of love that was sheer ecstasy. The love was so great, it was overpowering, yet comforting to me.* Beautiful,

beautiful dream. And I survived the night. Jean-Pierre never returned.

Jean-Pierre came creeping back to me the next day at the Palisades where I'd driven to limply and dumped my ashen body on the grass gasping for air. He was all over me, looking well rested and well f . .d. ''I'll help you'' he said, glancing around furtively to see if his new girlfriend was jogging by, and saw us together. I'd say I was hardly a threat in my condition; I needed a hospital; I didn't need him. Fortunately, for me, I was able to return to my house the following Wednesday.

Which brings me to the why of it all? What I found out at Jean-Pierre's was that I was full of fear — huge amounts — a direct sequelae of the disease, unacknowledged, even in my own heart. Physically, this left me very vulnerable. On my knees again, I surrendered my list of terrors to God — tar, roof materials, dying, paramedics picking me up good samaritanically and killing me with an IV or adrenalin preserved in phenol. The very next day, the life-threatening symptoms disappeared, as did the roofers. Once more, a peace flowed through me.

The neighbors had decided to repair the roof themselves: ''Let you know if we must use chemicals.'' But let me backtrack here.

Following the surrender of my fears of chemicals, another fear appeared: no place to go when they started the roof again. Jean-Pierre's keys represented life, while representing death. Too terrified to let them go, I hung on to them as my thread to life for as long as a week after I'd left his house without a goodbye.

An ''inner voice'' told me to return them. Despite great fear in my heart, courage drove me to his place. Opened the door, up the stairs, entered the bedroom, smelled the perfume, saw the pierced blue earrings on the night stand. With a pain in my heart, I dropped the keys on the bed, and walked out of his life. Four places to stay appeared the following day.

In the middle of all this madness, my nurse's aide informed me that termite pellets were all over the upstairs furniture and carpeting in various locations of the three bedrooms. Instead of becoming hysterical, I intrinsically knew all would turn out well. A phone call to the pesticide company brought rapid results. A serviceman came out and re-applied the electron gun, apologizing for the termites, saying the procedure was done as an emergency late at night when one can't see well. I believed him. The termite problem to this day, is caput.

A wonderful lesson came from this roof ordeal: I found out my body could tolerate a three day vacation at a nearby all electric hotel. And so it was revealed — I was more well than even I thought; that my isolation was truly over, and that it would take time to regain the confidence to enter life fully. But most of all I learned that I bounced back very rapidly from what would have destroyed me seven months ago. That was the miracle of the KIVA light.

* * * * * * * *

After I recovered from the roof poisoning, life began accelerating into more and more interesting paths. Paying a great deal of attention to my dreams clearly brought about a thread of cohesiveness to my recovery that had eluded me earlier. I had a series of dreams, for example, depicting me back in nursing school, only now as an undergraduate fearing she wouldn't complete school with her class due to a protracted illness. The first indication of this ''fear'' presented itself on December 22, 1983, . . . *in which I returned to nursing school after many years to re-register but I was so ill, I fainted at the registrar's desk . . . Next, I climbed up an elevator shaft to my old room which had been sealed after my departure . . . On my old bunkbed was a glass of milk and old food on a plate — about 20 years old . . . No one's been in this room since I left it . . . The window is a door . . . Outside it, I see grass blowing and then a sharp drop — a cliff . . . I look out into the hallway. All the other rooms are updated and the wallpaper is filled with green infinity signs; my room has blue ones, but it's very old . . . I don't have to worry about reacting . . . Comfortable. The environment is safe, not like outside (the cliff).*

My comprehension of the dream at that time was that the school was my body and the closed up room was my heart. The infinity signs gave me hope and assurance of healing while ensconced in this protected atmosphere. That was as much as I knew then.

The second dream in this series appeared right after the incident with Jean Pierre, whereby I returned his keys. *On June 9, I was back in nursing school . . . Had one more test to pass — math — but felt I couldn't do it . . . It was the last day of my training . . . That day I had to move my chest of drawers to a new apartment . . . A florist shop gives me a silver dolly to carry it . . . I start in my car for my apartment at 76th and Lexington in New York . . .*

Failing the math test meant to me that I still had some unknown fear I wouldn't heal completely. A chest of drawers possibly represented the emergence of a new female self. The silver carrier was heavenly support. Being on my way to my new apartment, I felt showed I wasn't quite healed yet. However, I did believe this dream revealed I'd completed another phase of my healing which was learning to love my self as a woman. (I'd always felt more masculine because I was strong — negative female conditioning in my childhood home).

That same night a third dream revealed even more progress. *Now, I was a patient at my old hospital, but was explaining to some visiting relatives that I'd been sick a lot and missed some of my schooling . . . It is May and I've finished nurse's training . . . While no one is looking, I escape from my hospital bed and go to the hospital's auditorium for a political meet-*

ing . . . However, when I walk in, a Mass is in progress . . . All my relatives are there . . . I kneel to pray and give thanks.

Obviously, this dream was telling me I was healed, but needed time to convalesce both physically and mentally after the acute life-threatening phase had ended. The escape from the hospital signified to me the end of my illness was near. My gratitude at the end, plus seeing what might be in store for my future (political involvement?), seemed to be guiding me to a new path in life.

The final dream on June 9 enlightened me as to how this all would come to fruition. *Amy (me at age 12) is getting out of the hospital . . . She dines in a dining room with her father (not real one) . . . I'm not invited to eat and feel very hurt, but sit down anyway and talk to them . . . They eat and leave. I go to the sink to wash my hands and see a yellow-green turd floating in the water . . . Then I see rats in a cage (or giant mice) . . . Two alive . . . Two dead on the floor . . . We put the dead ones in a cage and they revive . . . I think they are disgusting. Somehow, I think the rats are all dead . . . I open the cage door. One escapes . . . I chase it all over the table, but don't want to get bitten, so I don't touch it . . . The huge mouse (rat) runs into a small cage with no door . . . I put it up against the other cage so it can't escape . . . The piece of turd turned into one of the rats legs which I threw into the cage.*

Having some knowledge of what repeated symbols mean in my life by now, this dream brought to consciousness a lesson to be learned through lack. Rats or mice connote to me impoverishment of some kind. I had felt extreme lack, not only caused by the illness, but also catalyzed by losing Jean-Pierre's love, leaving a giant hole in my heart. Now that I was out of the hospital, a part of me (Amy) was ready with my God (the father), while the conscious part (adult Elizabeth) still had to learn some more lessons in order to be healed. The resurrection of the rat represented the Phoenix bird arising from the ashes to a new life in which I'd learned humility and proper use of my will. The final lesson in this dream was to place God as number one in my life, and the lack would disappear. Learning this lesson was the very toughest for me but, miraculously, completed my healing. Time would reveal when I'd ascended to this plateau.

The next step was — how do I find the way to let go of all lack? Standing right in front of me was the answer. Tom. It was he who had introduced me to the spiritual teacher, Sage King several months ago whom I've mentioned previously assisted me during my roof crisis. Sage seemed to be the next piece to the puzzle. Skeptical as hell of the kahuna's source of knowledge, and always looking for signs of guruitis, power and/or ego trips, I'd failed to discover any real objections to him in my observance of his Friday night classes. Then I had two dreams, telling me he was my next teacher. That clinched it for me. For by now, I knew the only method to heal me completely was to release from my body whatever was keeping me ill, in order to be freed forever of environmental illness. I was willing.

The results came fast. My second session proved to hold the key to my healing. For some reason, I mentioned to Sage that I'd had a frightening dream that Sunday. It went like this:

I'm in a clinic . . . They don't know how to treat my disease . . . I go into the kitchen and take a banana yogurt out of the refrigerator (I couldn't touch yogurt in real life) . . . I eat off the top layer and underneath is solid black petroleum . . . I am very scared . . . I look out my kitchen window — pitch black. All starts going black on me — I'm dying . . .

But I don't . . . I come to again, and a woman says that's what it feels like when you heal — at first you feel like you're dying.

I explained to Sage what I thought the dream meant: the banana topping was supposed to be my inner core which I was investigating; the petroleum — inner layers of my being or how I really saw myself; the woman — a spirit telling me I must die or let go of this negative inner core in order to live and heal.

Sage liked my interpretation. But he took it one step farther, which proved utterly fascinating. He said ''Let's dump the sludge out of the carton on a table.'' I visualized the scenario. ''What do you see?'' Joyfully, I replied, ''A glass bubble, a glass bubble is arising out of the black sludge.''

''Do you see a pearl?''

''No, just a glass bubble. And in it is a little girl, about 4 years old, wearing a child's white pinafore with blue trim. Surrounding her in the bubble is a brilliant, almost blinding golden light.''

''That is your spirit'' he shouted delightedly. ''That's how you came into this world. Now I want you to retain that image and practice meditating on it. That is the *real* you, Elizabeth.'' I broke down and cried, for my ignorance about *me* was gone, as I saw that I had believed myself black, bad — a degraded self-image which was entirely false. ''You are free,'' he went on. ''The illness will now heal itself, based upon the truth. That [the vision] is how God made you.''

Over the summer months, as a direct result of this session, I released tons of false ideas and unfounded guilts I had about myself which I'd formed on misinterpretations of childhood events. Granted, I'd truly had a disastrous childhood, but the self-image I'd formed was warped and untrue, and was based entirely on assumptions I'd made in reaction to my parents' destructive actions. Two months working with Sage consciously, and through dreams, freed me of past negative ideas which held tension in my body, thereby leaving me extremely vulnerable to serious illness.

The lessons I learned this summer with Sage are still in practice this very day. By August, I had learned all I could from him — now I had to incorporate this knowledge into my everyday life. I know I'll be at this for the rest of my life, because he opened the door to me as to how to stay healthy *after* you've healed the acute malady. In brief, an altered attitude toward oneself first, from negative to positive, and releasing the tension consciously in the body, is the key to recovery. The restoration of health follows as a natural progression of the body's ability to heal itself.

During my internship with Sage, another dream predicted my future. In this one, *I decide to go food shopping . . . The girls and I purchased a turkey . . . The counter men tell us they'll cook it for us . . . How long will the turkey take? . . . 117½ hours. We'll take rest of food home and come back for the turkey. Meanwhile, we stuff on popcorn . . . We go home to wait for the turkey.*

Turkey symbolizes autumn in my mind. Popcorn is a favorite binge food. Corn represents reaping a harvest. I took this to mean, that in September, I'd be well. Fantastic!

So when did the disease leave me? Well, let me add the final piece to this mosaic. On June 20, 1984, the finale came in a dream:

> *Dreamt admitted to the hospital . . . for a work up . . . refused all tests and medications . . . Nurse and doctor come in to do I.V.s and Foleys. They go to check me . . . I'm under the covers when a nurse comes in and gives me an injection in my right shoulder near my neck. I'm suffocating under the blankets . . . I fight her . . . What is that? . . . "Pabamine" . . . It's a cathartic and (can't remember) which makes you urinate . . . It has phenol — doesn't kill me . . . Tells me Demerol is ingredient. Drowsy . . . can't stay awake . . .*

The dream was telling me to let go of my old ideas about how sick I am — that the illness is over for me. I'm also being told to release it mentally because I won't have life-threatening reactions anymore. The dream revealed I carried a great deal of fear regarding the medical world harming me. *But nothing happens.* In fact, I am helped by the nurses and doctors.

As I awakened from this dream, my neck popped out of place. After getting my neck straightened by my chiropractor, I began experiencing tremendous anger. Pacing up and down the Palisades, I felt *something* was trapped in my body. I called Sage for help, but he was in a session. I went home and screamed angrily at everybody. Then I drove to a business appointment. On my way home, "something" made me put on a tape of the song, *Time* by Allan Parsons, saying goodbye to a lover. Was the pain Jean-Pierre? No, no response physically. Played the next number, Streisand singing the lead song from "Cats," *Memories. Midnight not a sound on the pavement* — a lament about letting go of someone and beginning a new life.

Pain shot up my insides as I burst into tears at the wheel of my car. In that moment, my gut released the illness and all the men I'd loved and been hurt by. My candidiasis-self died with my head bent over the wheel of the car. It was over. My love affair with death had died. I was free, free to start a whole new life, like a babe born free, pure, innocent and full of love. In that instant, I knew the disease had left me. Resurrection had begun. My whole life turned around that day, not beginning a new chapter, but a new book.

Several months later on Labor Day, I attended a party in Venice celebrating the coming together of a group of people dedicated to changing the world by placing love and humanity back into every field of endeavor. The afternoon was prolific — invited to speak at a local club and contacted a famous novelist's right-hand lady to interview me for a mind-brain newsletter. The interesting change I perceived in myself was: four months ago, freshly out of isolation and still reacting emotionally (fear) to my surroundings, I manifested toxic behavior — anger, paranoia and rage — plus symptoms of a person returning from long term trauma (isolation) — tearfulness, anger at any perceived put down, and fear of being asked what I did for a living. But Labor Day, all went well, for my illness induced emotional scars were healing as evidenced by my new behavior. For I was cheerful, smiling, friendly, and coherent. And even able to think about a career *of any kind*. That's when you know you've been healed.

Today as I close my story, life is becoming more and more beautiful. Off nystatin for good somewhere in February; using Pau only for colonics every week or so; watching my hair grow lighter and lighter chestnut every day, (and the white disappearing); color pink and vital; the 30 pounds gone from the nystatin; and only taking candida herbs occasionally (when I get reckless and binge on ice cream — Haagen Dazs vanilla — what else?) to protect myself from a reoccurrence — all mean a very visible health. At present, I'm experimenting with an herb named *Butcher's Broom* which allegedly clears up the damage to the arteries. Let me tell you — it really works and is very powerful, for I can feel pressure in my right shoulder and breastbone as if some "thing" were breaking up calcium deposits. Afterwards, leg and kidney aching ensues. A very powerful detoxer for the entire cardiovascular system. One a week is enough for me, otherwise I become too tired to function. Vitamin C can also now be tolerated without any side effects. Energy is boundless; only cantaloupe and sugar remain taboo (although I cheat occasionally on the sugar part). And my KIVA light remains in my kitchen doing its quiet job.

My children are blossoming, grateful this horror is over. Amy wants to be an orthopedic surgeon, Jen an artist: both will have the guidance and nurturing from me they'll need now that I am functioning. As for me, a writing career is in full bloom out of my home; a lecturing one — on candidiasis — is in its infancy. The major poisonous chemicals — paint, tar and formaldehyde — are not used in my home. The girls have been able to use normal shampoo and conditioners since June without affecting me. And greatest of all, I washed my hair last week for the first time with a naturally scented shampoo and accompanying protein conditioner (I'd used avocadoes pureed for the past year to oil my dried-out hair) — that truly is a miracle. But the most fun of all is that I ate pizza (cheese!) two weeks ago and *nothing happened*.

Orie claims the nervous system takes eighteen months to heal with his lights; I say I'll be fully healed this September — 1984. We'll see who's right.

Tom. You ask what happened to Tom? Ah. Well. We're still so busy helping one another re-enter life, I don't have time to talk about it. Why, that's a whole other book too.

To fully demonstrate how far I've really come, let me close my tale with the final dream in the nursing school series. On the night of September 18th my birthday, I dreamt *I returned to nursing school once more to complete the 3 year course . . . In this particular dream, my class was graduating in September [now] . . . I'm very sad because I've missed most of my second year . . . Don't know if I'll ever make it [to graduate] . . . Then, I remember I am an R.N. and rush into the nurse's residence. All my former classmates are there smiling at me . . . They haven't changed in all these years . . . All [I believed back then] were much more secure than I . . . I run up a long flight of wooden stairs . . . As I reach the top, I spill my cup of coffee (or milk) all over the staircase and on someone's sandwich sitting below me . . . The cup runs over and spills down through the stairs . . . A real naughty! I laugh joyously at myself and get paper towels to clean it up . . . Everyone smiles at me again . . . Earlier in this segment, I was in a large auditorium with my class . . . I was laughing at the absurdity of my worrying about finishing school . . . Here, I realized my entire class had one more year to study too . . . I was relieved . . . I wasn't so far behind, or alone.*

The kahuna had told me earlier when the emotional body healed, the physical would follow. His wisdom seemed proven by this dream. For I felt it meant the acute life-threatening phase was completely over *along with* the emotional baggage of my past that had helped to create it. The year's further study told me it would be another year before my body, mind, and heart completely mended. That heartened me, for I knew there has to be a long period of reconstruction *after* the acute phase of the illness subsides in which the body remains somewhat vulnerable while healing. But especially difficult is the mending of the emotional scars of re-facing life, a drop at a time, chemical by chemical (over 2000 of them) with nothing happening. Only a year to get on my feet completely — why that would be wonderful — and a miracle. And I'd have a lot of help doing it (the spirit of my classmates) from compassionate, loving people.

The cup running over symbolized my gratitude for "graduating." Suddenly, it dawned on me as I re-read this vision, that I had graduated from the "school of learning-to-heal-yourself," and nursing school was only a symbol. Why, Jesus took three years to complete his ministry and passion. Was there a spiritual connection? And three years was the length of nursing school training and my illness. The irony here seemed to be three years was the magical course, *if you learned your lessons.* I believe I did.

Now, all I had to do was go out and put into practice what I had learned. Easier said than done. For healing the brutal beating my body had taken and re-entering life as a whole person were quite a stiff order. But another challenge to be met. Another plateau, another graduation — and then what? Life had become once more, an unending adventure.

This book would not be complete if I didn't inform you that the healing of systemic candidiasis is manifold. No doctor, drug, therapist, or person can do it for you. Recovery requires taking charge of your own illness by changing your attitude or belief system from negativity, to positive speech and thought patterns, by making a conscious decision to be well, and by doing the action necessary to being about the desired result — health, happiness and prosperity. Not easy, but worth it, as you will see as we go on. For the key to healing is to restore the body's natural balance. Balance comes through the tools in the following chapters.

PART III

THE HEALING

MENTAL HEALING

I suppose by now you wonder how I stayed sane through all this. Sane, I remained. The techniques I used to transcend my sense of isolation and abandonment were simple, loving, and *daily*. For one isn't greeted with much sympathy with this condition. There are consistently several reactions by fellow humans — fear, avoidance, all-in-your-head cliches and abandonment. Ninety-nine percent of EI's are abandoned by spouses, lovers, friends, and families. A tragic statistic — but I speak from experience. Therefore,it is essential not to abandon yourself. In order to survive and heal without abandoning oneself, self-love is a must. Loving myself required building up my self-esteem, then letting go of the fears within.

Fear, as you know by now, becomes one's constant companion in E.I. Terrifying, unmitigated fear. Lovelessness. It is the sequelae of having a poisoned body and mind that turns on you without notice. A feeling of being out of control; powerlessness develops. One regresses to a childish, even infantile state of mentality which is a natural result of prolonged, devastating illness. Life is no longer life, but a daily challenge to survive in an environment that has transformed itself into a palpable nightmare. No touching, no human contact, no control over the body's reacting on *whichever chemical assaults it.*

Along with the devastating physical and emotional sequalae, the E.I. develops a ''toxic personality.'' Brain toxicity produces many universal symptoms: phobias, obsessive-compulsive thinking, paranoia, negativity, anger, depression, suicidal ideation, violent rage out of nowhere, extreme agitation and hostility. These symptoms are physiologically produced; ''it'' is not the person's true self. This distinction is necessary here, for candidiasis sufferers are judged by society in general on the surface personality. The sufferer notices the personality change but eventually forgets what he or she was originally like. As the disease progresses, the victim can no longer distinguish between what is him and what is the disease. Tragic, for the victims start believing the reactions are them.

To illustrate this point more clearly, I'll include Tom's comments on my "personality changes" since he met me last September, and the present September.

"You know Elizabeth, your attitude improved a 1000% since I met you last year, and a 100% since the last party I took you to in March."

"What do you mean?" I asked edgily, thinking I was being judged again as the disease.

"Well, now you're loving, cheerful, friendly and open to meeting people. The last time you were hostile and angry."

"Yes Tom," I explained (one even has to clarify who they are *with a fellow victim* for they too, have forgotten who they were, and usually didn't know you before the disease). "A year ago, I had fresh toxic poisoning from pesticides. In March, I was reacting emotionally more than physically to the stress of a new environment. Two years of isolation produces a complete fear of life. The physical was healed, but my emotions weren't. I was terribly fragile then. I wasn't like this before the illness."

Lovingly, he said "Elizabeth, think about putting this in your book. It's very important — the lack of control over the personality change."

Yes Tom, it is extremely important, for this combination of physical and mental alterations which are intensified by stress, whether physical or emotional, leaves the candidiasis sufferer with a terrifying feeling of powerlessness.

Therefore, powerlessness is the main mental characteristic of the yeast victim. The environment can be controlled up to a point; it cannot be totally controlled to provide a healthy, functional life. From this powerlessness erupts an intense feeling of isolation and deprivation — and complete terror of all chemicals. Serious illness, isolation, severe human deprivation, no support from society: the set up is for suicide.

Needless to say, the answer lies within yourself in these circumstances to survive: this is the greatest challenge of candidiasis. For no illness on earth, in my cognizance, produces such intense hopelessness and isolation from human comfort. Human love and comfort is essential to the well being of the organism. We are severed from this sustenance. Then how do we endure? The solution comes from within our own hearts.

The brutal way I was first diagnosed left me panic stricken and reeling mentally. *I couldn't be that sick. Allergic to everything in the 20th Century!* The doctor must be insane. Unfortunately, he wasn't. But I almost went insane hearing what was wrong with me. All those years of going from doctor to doctor — "We don't know what's wrong" kept ringing in my ears in unison. Being thought psychotic, neurotic, or emotionally distraught, i.e. an anxiety reaction. Yes, I was distraught — about their diagnoses.

Still, when one hears the ramifications of E.I. in detail, the only response is shock, fear and panic. Also denial. And you already have a creeping nameless fear building up stronger and stronger everyday, that you don't dare to admit even to yourself. Yet, the diagnosis provided a reason, the why, which I needed to know, shocking as it was. My worst fears were verified; I was dying.

The nurse, a sufferer herself, ran the litany of chemicals, foods, and substances I needed to remove from my home in order to survive. *Blurred mouth, running like a motor . . . Mind shuts down, screaming, shut up, I can't stand anymore . . . Falling out the door, driving home blind with fear . . . the scream inside me erupted when I picked up the phone to tell someone . . . anyone the truth — they'd found out what was wrong with me, and I was going to die from the knowledge . . .*

If you survive this stage, you're on your way to getting well. Breaking down further each day, while being told how seriously ill you are, is a bonafide nightmare. Especially in my case, living in a brand new city alone with two young children, knowing absolutely no one. Well, not quite that bad — I did go out of my way to make acquaintances before I made the permanent move to prevent this isolation. The best plans of mice and men can go astray. Not only did they go astray, they were bludgeoned to death. Normal answers to ordinary life processes do not apply with E.I.

To survive, I reached backwards to Jean-Pierre's hand, telling myself this was staying alive. As much as I disliked him and wanted to let him go, I needed his kind side to make it. At this point in time, I realized it was important not to let go of any human contact, no matter how limited, while telling myself this was necessary for survival. It took me a long time to get realistic and stop beating myself up for this choice. Since I'd been a beauty with my choice of good men, this required rapid ego deflation. *Take the crumbs now, the cake will follow when you are well.* Many times a day, I had to remind myself of that fact. Many. For the brain toxicity takes over in reactions causing you to view negatively any life-saving decision you made previously. Therefore, I found it necessary to write these truths down, tacking them within eyeshot, so I had instant reference to them, no matter what condition I was in.

And there were times, many in fact, whereby my brain was too insane to execute even these simple tools. There's where the true challenge came in. Several solutions occurred to me. Set up a network, people you can call in emergencies (put a cotton washcloth over the phone if plastic is intolerable). Fellow E.I.s, old friends, therapists, new acquaintances. Train them. Tell them exactly what happens to you when a reaction occurs. Have them write down a list of your needs at this time and read them back to you when you're in a reaction. Verbal affirmation, ''This is only chemical,'' has a very soothing effect. You don't have to explain anything; they already know. No one in a reaction is emotionally prepared to start explaining the problem to anyone. I emphasize, *teach them beforehand.* Comprise a list like this:

1) Tell me I'm in a chemical reaction (I may not even know it, but one's voice clearly changes to a knowing friend).
2) Tell me ''Hang in there, it will pass.''
3) This is most important — tell the caller not to discuss the madness you are spewing forth — it's chemical poisoning — but to reinforce over and over to the sufferer its chemical nature — it will pass.
4) Have the person read to you the list of items that will alleviate the reaction:

    a) Leave the area if necessary
    b) Close the windows if applicable (or open them).
    c) Use oxygen for the anoxia (lack of oxygen to the brain).
    d) Immunplex or alka seltzer, or salts to stop the reaction (whichever works for you).
    e) Turn on electric heaters if it's mold and sit right next to them — heat kills mold.
    f)) take a shower, change clothes, go to clean air — showers remove positive ions from the body affording some relief.
    g) If you can't help yourself at all, instruct them to talk kindly and lovingly to you, no matter what you are saying.

The important fact here is love. Let others love you when you are unable to love yourself. The healing can be miraculous. *We do need people.* We must learn to take what they can offer. Our needy state drives others away after awhile. That is a cruel fact of life.

To avoid abandonment as much as possible, it's important to rotate your phone calls to your supporters, otherwise they will burn out. No one individual can handle all the ramifications of E.I. *No one.* For those of you who have been deserted and are alone, there is a Reaction Hotline in Berkeley, California (415-644-1400) where you will be listened to by compassionate volunteers. Some E.I.'s argue, ''I can't afford the call.'' My argument is, if your life is on the line, make the call and worry about the bill afterwards. Until a national network is set up, this is all we have.

Use the phone for another purpose too — to bring the world *into* you. When one is not ill, and those times do exist, call friends, inquire about their daily life, ask about movies, plays, books they've read. *Get out of yourself!* Endlessly talking about being ill will pull you down. Avoid listening to anyone's problems as much as you can — *this is self-preservation.* The same applies for people living with you. Have them bring the outside world to you. Participate as much as possible in ordinary life even if it means listening to a child or spouse, half-conscious. *It will keep you sane.* Moving to a community with all E.I.'s would have ended my sanity. For me not to go mad, I had to surround myself with some healthy people. Other E.I.'s were helpful when I needed to hear a voice who understood my plight.

However, be sure not to lean on fellow E.I.'s too heavily; they are sufferers too and have limits. I learned this early on. If a kind E.I. would listen to my suicidal depressions and didn't sound in a reaction herself, I'd go full volume. Of course, I was too toxic to realize her position — this is a very sad part of our particular illness. Obsessional thinking will turn people off after awhile, due to their feelings of helplessness in the situation. Again, I emphasize, teach your listener. In this way you'll save yourself a lot a heartache and further abandonment.

For abandonment and excruciating loneliness are two of the major mental problems one has to deal with in E.I.

Let's take abandonment first. Ninety-nine percent of E.I.'s are deserted by spouses and family. Strangely enough, in my multi-experiences talking with the seriously ill, they come from homes where emotional abandonment was a usual pattern by their parents. This was true in my case. On the other hand, some others did not experience this desertion, but did have loving families that did support and love them through this initiation into hellfire; they heal faster. However, I've found this to be the exception rather than the rule.

Having no emotional tools to deal with abandonment, I had to learn new methods to cope with this severe pain. One of them was writing. Day by day, in my lonely ''cell,'' I wrote out the pain, the fear, the anger and the dread of dying alone. At the same time, I chronicled my progress — up or down, in or out. To me it was forward, no matter what happened, because I had some answers to my dilemma. This brought a balance to my life that had a healing effect. Through writing, I put my pain out there on paper while succeeding in encouraging myself to get well. This daily releasing of the emotional stress saved my sanity.

No matter what shape I was in, I scribbled down something each day about getting well. Putting the pain ''out there'' also dilutes the intensity. Lastly, I worked an intense spiritual program which I'll get into in detail in the next chapter.

Crying is a wonderful healing tool to deal with loneliness and abandonment; sharing it with a compassionate person heals one even faster. Tears, most times, were my only solace in the early days of my confinement. For no one understood what I was going through — no one. Not my therapist, nor some fellow E.I.'s — most had never been this sick. Rejection by them was the most painful, but it happened. This intensified the feelings of loneliness and isolation. So, crying was a major source of survival initially.

Rage was another survival tool. I raved at God, mankind and my friends about why could this happen to me. What kind of Creator could allow such an abomination? The powerlessness was overwhelming; the rage was eternal. But constantly raging breaks the body down further; it also releases old trapped energy one isn't in touch with: I had to use it in moderation when appropriate, when I wasn't out of control, raving in a chemical reaction. If this all sounds terribly calm, it wasn't. Just continuous, tough, logical decisions to remain sane. For without one's sanity, one could not survive E.I. For I've seen the unfortunates who didn't get help, who stayed angry and bitter. One day,they crossed a fine line permanently into brain toxicity. I weep for them for they are so hard to reach.

Seeing this tragedy made me even more determined not to wind up that way. Yes, I had brain toxicity, among other symptoms; no, I refused to become that way. A quest for health became my god.

Finding a mentor is very helpful. Eve was my main teacher in the very critical phase. Her warmth and compassion helped me. But most of all, her knowledge gave me hope. Only one other E.I. I spoke to was getting well; the rest were bitter and angry, hating doctors, chemical companies and the world in general. Although I couldn't blame them, I also didn't want to join that line of thinking. There was no deliberate plot to make we human beings this ill. It just was. A product of technology misused. To me, we had to take responsibility for our own health, heal first, then educate the masses. I set that goal for myself, as had Eve.

Goal setting is a terrific way to offset the emotional devastation. And they must be small at first. And realistic. If you are recovering from total isolation with life-threatening symptoms, you don't run out to a high school graduation filled with cigarette smoke as your first outing (like I did). No, you make it simple.

For instance, go for a walk. If it's 10 minutes — great, if it's 5 seconds, congratulate yourself for leaving the house for that amount of time. Make the smallest step forward a mountain. Make the biggest step backwards a lesson. Give yourself credit for standing up that day if you couldn't get off your bed before then.

The goals must be small, realistic and enhance your self-esteem in the early healing. These are short term goals. Long term goals give you something to look forward to. I, for instance, fantasized a trip to Europe, visualizing medieval castles of Scotland, rivers and mountains in Switzerland, and interesting people. On a more practical plane, I planned attending my daughter Jen's 8th grade graduation. Which I did. Which also brought on a severe reaction from cigarette smoke, whereby I collapsed, turning my lovely shade of gray again. No matter, I went. That was the important part. Let go of the negative, focus on the success. In other words, focus on the goal — recovery; live through the obstacles — reactions. The healing will take leaps and bounds with this attitude.

Support groups are another helpful tool. We formed one in Berkeley, but it was sadly comical: one E.I. asked for the windows to be shut because she developed severe chest pain from woodsmoke; one asked they be open as she reacted on the rug; one sniffed the couch and felt like vomiting; I went through shaking chills no matter what they did. The group setting can be very beneficial depending on who runs it. If it focuses on self-pity and depression, all go away drained. If it focuses on how we can help ourselves, the group energy is healing. Yet as you can see, most E.I.'s in my condition can attend nothing. So we need other solutions.

Recently, I started a meeting by mail. Being in its infancy, I don't know the outcome at present. What I do know is the idea was met with enthusiasm by several sufferers in different cities nationwide. Communication of any kind is a life saver for people locked in their cage at home, seeing and touching no one. Life saving in the sense that they don't commit suicide from despair in their torment. These people who have been abandoned by life for so long hardly believe there's any love out there, no matter who sends it. That is why I believe it is especially important to help one another. A post card, a kind word, words of encouragement. One sentence. ''I love you'' — one sentence may save a life. Anyone who wishes to help can contact me. However, let me make this perfectly clear: there is no obligation, no pressure, only a desire to have human contact, and the desire to write, even one line, when one is able. That's it. A lifeline.

Another ''outside'' aid, or external tool is finding people to hug and hold you. Usually, ''mold people'' are limited to one another, that is the ones who can get around and meet others. The tragedy here is we usually cannot ''tolerate'' one another. In my own experience, I attempted to start a loving relationship with a very humorous male E.I. of 28. Getting to his home in San Francisco from mine in Berkeley took almost all I had mentally and physically, for I had to survive the car fumes on the Oakland Bay Bridge. Prior to this development, we'd kept one another sane by laughing uproariously at the absurdity of our situation by phone.

Joseph could use a skin moisturizer and a scented soap; I couldn't. The plan was to stay for the weekend, to enjoy one another, to have some play. It didn't work out that way. He couldn't cook indoors at all or use anything beyond a 25 watt bulb in his house, or his entire body turned bright red, burning like fire, followed by anaphylactic shock. This proved very stressful for me who could do these things, and became even more limited trying not to harm him while I was there, while simultaneously hoping not to go down from the added stresses myself. One thing led to another and we wound up in bed together. His moisturizer and toxic mattress sent me into cerebrals and exhaustion; my shampoo and body odor made him collapse. Sadly, nothing happened. Devastating for him, who cried ''If I'm impotent from this disease too, I'll kill myself.'' Me, filled with mad voices and sympathy, held him. Nausea and triple vision besieged me. Depressing. In total despair, we both eventually slept.

When I left the next day, we both knew it wasn't meant to be. There was nothing to say or cry over, for I had to save every ounce of energy to make it back across that bridge. Leaving one another was terribly painful. Joseph looked abandoned. My only thought was self-preservation. The trip across the bridge (yes I made it) resulted in suicidal depressions. Jean-Pierre happened to be in Palo Alto visiting his almost ex-wife and children. Letting go of revenge, I phoned him, crying with despair about my situation, telling him I wanted to commit suicide, and making him feel awful for not being with me. Actually, I wanted to kill him, but decided to use him instead, for guilt worked very well with Jean-Pierre. He offered to come pick me up and fly me back to L.A. with him — a very unrealistic solution. Defeated, I hung up on him. The cerebral passed. So did my despair.

But I didn't give up completely on getting touched. A few months later, I tried again, this time with a brilliant E.I. living way out by the Pacific Ocean. Dosed on nystatin about two months, but unable to drive myself, I had Kevin pick me up and take me to his house. He was intelligent, uplifting company. Very easy to be with. An attempt at lovemaking was abortive, again. When he came near my body, I lapsed into exhaustion. There is a belief among E.I.'s that we react off the mold spores on one another's bodies. I tend to believe this.

Which leads me to why I said, don't let go of anyone, not even the crumbs. Jean-Pierre was totally willing to use no hair spray, no conditioner, unscented shampoo, olive oil soap, and wear cotton clothes washed in Erlander's washing soda. Could I let go of that? No, for through him, I could depend on getting hugs, kisses, and loving once a month, sometimes more often. No way would I give this up. For in my mind, I had decreed that this illness was analogous to being in a concentration camp; the illness represented the camp, the continuous reactions, Hitler. Our bodies had become our own torture machine, never knowing when, where or how the torture would begin.

In order to survive my own body's betrayal, I had to take love where I could find it, no matter how imperfect: Jean-Pierre fit the bill. So I mentally blocked out his dark side and enjoyed his lighted side. Had I allowed myself to think or feel how I truly felt towards him, I may have murdered him. When one is this sick and isolated, with a body tortured by pain and madness, anything is possible, for this disease brings chronic high stress.

Which brings me to a very important survival tool: *Not thinking*. To survive E.I. at this desperate stage, one must wear blinders, looking straight ahead, no matter what. Never lose sight of the goal — wellness. Ignoring negative people and negative situations at first is difficult, but when your body goes into shock from the stress, you realize this stress is literally killing you. It was a great lesson in learning what's important in life — living. One can't live if they are dead. It became that simple for me. I said the healing was simple, but definitely not easy. Immediately turning a negative thought into a positive one *consciously*, stopped me from *beginning* reactions. When the movers showed up, for instance, full of cigarette smoke on their shirts causing me to go into shock the day before I left Berkeley, this little mental trick saved my life. Not focusing on what they did in their ignorance, to harm me (when I recovered of course), but zeroing in on my goal — to get to Santa Monica alive — I was able to let go of my rage at them. *Letting go is self-love;* it's the only way to get well. Releasing my emotional pain gave me abundant energy to direct the move — from my bed. For petty trivia are the trials in life that make us all angry and upset. Learning to let go of that perfectionism leaves the body plenty of energy to heal. I know — I did it.

One more important tool in enduring E.I. is the plain old daily calendar. On my wall in another room, hung a giant calendar. On it, I marked ''good day,'' ''bad day.'' As time went on the good days were longer and longer, the bad fewer and fewer. Whenever I felt set back or despairing of ever being well, I looked at the calendar which verified for me the ''good days'' were more often than the bad. It stamps that picture indelibly in the brain, that you are progressing forward, even if you are in a cerebral. Eventually the calendar was written in green crayon pens for ''good days'' while black marked the bad. Finally, I reached 95% good days. The other days, were more like normal life — an occasional flu or minor ailment — the afflictions of *ordinary* people. *It's important not to strive for perfection, only progress.* Self-esteem continues to be enhanced by these external tools.

Another powerful external aid is self-hypnosis or meditation tapes. For clarity, I'll only discuss self-hypnosis with the reader. Meditation will be elaborated on in the next chapter. Dr. Cort attempted hypnotizing me — I didn't like that. Someone else controlling my mind frightened me. However, Sherry provided me with an acceptable form — self-hypnosis tapes. In my understanding, self-hypnosis is only a means of talking directly to your subconscious. As skeptical as I was, remembering childhood ideas of occultism and grade-B movies with Svengali-types hypnotizing people and making them their slaves, and with great trepidation, I decided to try it. Surprisingly her relaxation tape worked wonders. (By the time she opened me up to this, I could ''tolerate'' tape recorders again.) Being afraid to use adrenalin for anaphylaxis, this new instrument provided me with an alternative to fear, panic and death.

The tape consisted of a gentle voice teaching me deep breathing and releasing the air from far inside my lungs. E.I.'s are shallow breathers genetically, I suppose. Hence, the oxygenation of the blood stream and brain are faulty to begin with. The breathing techniques reduced the reactions markedly; they likewise reduced the fear and panic. As the soft voice continued, she instructed you to bring light through your body: peace was the result. From that day forward, the self-hypnosis tape alleviated a great deal of my suffering. Today I know more advanced, powerful techniques, but that's getting ahead of myself again.

To remove a great deal of stress during acute episodes, in which you are relatively helpless, physically and mentally, it is wise to prepare beforehand, in a non-reaction, a list of your basic needs:

How and what foods to prepare.

What you can drink.

Any supplements that assist recovery.

The dosage and times of your nystatin or herbs.

Tag this on the refrigerator where last minute aides or family can see what needs to be done. If you have no one, this will prevent you from O.D.-ing on nystatin or any other supplement because you can't remember whether you took it or not. Once more, I remind you, there are times when even these tools fail. However, resolutions to that dilemma will be provided shortly. Keep on going, there is hope.

A finely tuned psychologist is another potent helper. One of mine, Sherry, was oriented towards meditation and breathing, along with talk; the other, Zena, gave love and support to my suffering, despite not completely understanding the disease. She listened. The key to a therapist truly assisting you is finding one who *really listens.* Fortunately, both of these women were open. Once, I had to scream at Sherry because I was reacting during a session on the mold in her house, in which agitation and fear were the manifestations. Sherry compassionately tried to treat ''it'' as emotional. The frustration of explaining to a fellow E.I. that the symptoms are chemically induced produces more anger. But it is important to speak up and trust yourself. *A reaction is a reaction. An emotion is an emotion.* The former is physically exteriorily induced; the latter interiorly produced: both appear identical on the surface.

That's why I feel it's important to find a compassionate therapist and educate them about the disease. In that way, you gain self-respect and theirs. If you allow yourself to be badgered by who *they* think you are, you'll leave a session depressed and even feeling more abandoned. *It's very, very important to believe in yourself.* Strength will appear to fortify you, through educating yourself on the ailment, and bringing articles and books to the therapist, if necessary. But remember, no counselor is perfect. They misunderstand and misinterpret. The hardest problem to deal with in oneself is the overwhelming anger and rage at not being understood. A good therapist can permit you to get angry and stand up for yourself. Look for these characteristics.

Sherry taught me one beautiful thing: whenever Jean-Pierre visited and left me after our weekend together, to treat myself like a baby for 3 or 4 days. A seriously ill person feels abandoned if someone they love goes away, even for a day. Kindness to oneself helps heal this very *real* wound. Wrestling alone with these feelings, made me feel less than human, resulting in beating myself up emotionally. With her suggestion, I saw a new way. Instead of avoiding feeling abandoned, I acknowledged it, then went on to write out what I could do to give myself pleasure. It worked. The cut healed, the pain diluted, then disappeared.

Next, I focused on what was right in my life, no matter how small. This, too, will keep one's sanity. Tell yourself, ''This too shall pass. I will be well. This is temporary. There is an answer. Help will come.'' In this way, you'll give yourself hope when no one else is handing it to you. So much of the healing is inside ourselves.

Which brings me to our next segment, the ''inside'' tools — the most powerful healer for candidiasis.

THE SPIRITUAL HEALING

Before you skip this chapter, let me make clear this is not a lecture on religion. Not at all. My definition of spiritual is the pragmatic use of one's own inner resources to bring about the desired result: recovery.

Forgiveness is the most formidable spiritual technique. Through letting go of resentments and bitterness toward any person, place or thing — the body heals. I outlined a 12-step program based on AA, that teaches unconditional love, which worked in every circumstance of my life. These guidelines were taught by me in our little support group:

1) We admitted we were powerless over chemicals — that our life had become unmanageable.
2) Came to believe that a Power greater than ourselves could restore us to sanity from the brain toxicity.
3) Made a decision to turn our will and our lives over to the care of God, *as we understood Him.*
4) Made a searching and fearless moral inventory of ourselves.
5) Admitted to ourselves, and to another human being the nature of our faults, then surrendering them to a Higher Power.
6) From this inventory, made a list of our character defects.
7) Humbly ask our Higher Power to remove these defects of character.
8) Made a list of people to whom we owed amends.
9) Made amends without bringing harm to ourselves or *anyone* else.
10) Took a daily inventory of assets and liabilities to keep ourselves balanced, immediately forgiving ourselves for wrong actions, and asking assistance to strengthen us while crediting ourselves for loving actions.

11) Sought through prayer and meditation a conscious contact with God.

12) Having had a spiritual awakening as a result of these steps, we tried to carry the message to other candidiasis sufferers, and to practice these principles in all our affairs.

The 12 steps are suggestions only. Through them, I found self-love. However, in my experience, by practicing these principles on a daily basis in every area of my life, I came to understand the meaning of unconditional love; it is love without expectations placed on any person, place or thing; it is giving without wanting; it is loving an unloveable person as a fellow human being. This does not mean we allow ourselves to be abused or hang around abusive people. No. Not at all. It is the deep, abiding love the Creator has for us and wishes us to experience; it is an ideal. Progress is all we can expect, not perfection. Learning to love ourselves unconditionally, frees us from fear, and allows us to heal, live, and receive abundance, as life was meant to be.

Self-love requires a great deal of *healthy* selfishness when you are so ill; *self love comes through forgiveness.* Taking action, working these steps, was how I achieved and still am achieving, my recovery.

The first three steps I say daily as soon as I awaken. That starts my day off on a positive, peaceful note. This did not happen overnight. Trial and error, laziness and non-belief, led me on a slow path. Having been an atheist, I was a tough nut to crack. Becoming critically ill *forced* me to work these steps, for I wouldn't have survived without them — my case was too far gone. Before I had these tools, I believed totally in self-reliance and super-independence. My life unmanageable? As long as I could work and support myself, I needed no outside help. I spit in my Higher Power's face for the past eighteen years of my life. At every opportunity, I crucified verbally anyone who believed in God. Weaklings. Need to believe some invisible source is helping them. Good for the masses. Gives them hope. Not me, I'm too self-sufficient. Well, Miss Self-Sufficient was brought to her knees by chemical toxicity, in fact, flat on her face on the floor, yelling ''If there is a God, *help me.*'' In these instances, a flood of warmth flowed through my body — the anaphylaxis ceased. Truly, I was amazed.

I am powerless over chemicals. Yes, my body was beaten by chemicals. I could not control every chemical in the environment. It was beyond human capability. Admitting I was powerless over chemicals allowed me to let go of a great deal of fear, thereby permitting my body to relax and heal. Fighting the effect of chemicals on my body served to increase the severity of the reaction. I told myself there must be something to this.

It was through these experiences that I became teachable, finding that self-reliance had limits while reliance on a Higher Power brought limitless possibilities. The unmanageability of my life was that I did not manage the universe. When I fully understood the second half of the first step, a comfort developed inside me, knowing I could fully depend on a power outside myself. That's true power.

The second step surrenders the brain toxicity to a Higher Power. It is necessary to practice this step *prior* to a reaction so that you can easily turn it over to God when a reaction hits you. Eventually some spark of brain clarity ensues, giving you hope that one day you will have comnand of your own mind again. This particular step saved my sanity when I couldn't separate the chemical reaction from my core being *and* healed old twisted thinking simultaneously.

Poppycock you say. Well, Herbert Spencer said ". . .condemnation prior to investigation . . . keeps a man in everlasting ignorance." Humbled, I acknowledged my ignorance.

Humiliation had been my idea of humility. The suffering, rejection, dehumanization and despair of E.I. had brought multiple humiliations into my life. Miss Independent couldn't work, couldn't start a business, couldn't complete a sentence, couldn't remember appointments, couldn't rear her children, couldn't keep an intimate relationship going, couldn't be depended on to show up for a date; *I was not this way before I became so ill.* Prior to the illness, having had my choice of men led to, during the illness, being *chosen* for a one night stand, that is, *if* you could function. Although I never succumbed to these advances by men, I felt emotionally humiliated and degraded by my powerless situation. Perhaps humiliation taught me to take another look at humility.

True humility began when I surrendered my life and will to a power higher than myself. True power developed from admitting the powerlessness of my situation. The third step taught me to let go of controlling the disease and learning to master it. Control takes a lot of energy, devitalizing the body. Mastery surrenders control, freeing more and more energy for healing. Surrender removes separation from the Source of all Light (energy). Surrender removes self-abandonment, as one becomes *powerful* through attaching to the source of all power — God.

Humbleness is not a key word in 1985. Arrogance has replaced it. In order to be humble, one must let go of thinking they are the center of the universe. E.I. forces one into self-centered fear, an abandoned child's state. The steps taught me the way out, through love.

Call a Higher Power what you will, I chose Love or God. Either suits me. "Charlie" or "Tree" may suit you. For those who can't or won't believe, a candidiasis support group can be your Higher Power. In any event, love is the great healer, and arrogance is the great stealer. Without love, I've not seen much recovery with E.I.; with it, I've experienced miracles.

Self-love begins with baby steps. Over and over, I told myself "I am worthwhile breathing" when I wasn't able to get off my bed. This baby step was the beginning of self-esteem. Deliberately, I overlooked all that was negative in my life (almost everything was) and focused on what I could do (which wasn't much).

"I stood up today. I fed myself. I cooked my own food. I opened the front door without collapsing." Sounds silly? Not at all. Spiritual progress is slow, step upon step, building up the destroyed self-esteem. "I'm worthwhile breathing" proved the most beneficial worth builder as I spent many days virtually functionless, needing to be cared for like a baby, without parents to tend me. *Devastating.* Being alone, with the exception of two young children who do not take care of you (they can help some, but this disease is overwhelming for a mature adult). Having no husband or friends to help me forced me to reach inside myself for something more powerful than myself. For without a Higher Power, I was doomed. Never would I have been humbled sufficiently without being fatally ill, to reach out for a Creator. This I did. It's the only reason I'm alive today. Ask the doctors who saw my case.

With the working of the third step also came the knowledge that one's reaction can be used to bring about healing. For behind the rage, paranoia, insanity and suicidal depressions, hid some genuine repressed feelings. By surrendering my cerebrals to a Higher Power, a peace entered my being. Simultaneously, I became more and more aware of old beliefs about myself that weren't true. Abandonment was the biggest lie about myself to myself, that I discovered. Crying out my rage at God enlightened me that I'd believed since childhood my parents *always* abandoned me emotionally when the truth was they didn't know what to do. It was only a belief, but a destructive one, destroying my self-esteem. When I let go of this false idea (after a reaction), some form of healing always followed.

The 4th and 5th steps are to teach us honesty about ourselves. Done properly, this gives one a balance as to who one is, positive and negative. Some people think they're perfect; others feel they are worthless: neither attitude permits growth. Healing can only take place in an open mind. Since E.I.s are "mindless" during cerebrals, we must focus on learning self-love, *when we are clear*. If there are continuous cerebrals, there are other methods which I'll get into later.

I wrote a 4th step when I was dying in October '81 in Berkeley. The guilt and anger I still carried with me surprised even me. A 4th step is just listing persons, places or things one resents and listing the reason you feel this way, then how it affects you emotionally. Here are several examples:

Resentment	*Cause*	*Affects*
father	drunk and beat me	hated him and self (self-esteem)
mother	teaching me by example women are doormats	angry for being female (lowers self-esteem)
Jean-Pierre	cruel to me	feels I'm unloveable (destroys self-esteem)

The fifth step is sharing the fourth step with someone you trust, who understands your purpose is life and death. Any compassionate soul will do, or a fellow E.I. who's already done this. After sharing my story with a Catholic priest, the continuous anaphylactic reactions stopped and became less and less in frequency.

Obviously, I hadn't cleared out all the old wreckage of the past, but it was a beginning. An inventory is like peeling layers off an onion. Each time you do one, more and more is released, more and more healing takes place. There was such a history of abuse in my background that I only did what was at the surface in my mind. Digging into myself would have made me crack up — there was just too much inside me. (Each year, I'd do a thorough inventory.) I deal with the garbage as it comes up now.

After reading the 5th step to my trusted friend, I went off by myself and reviewed what I had done. Then I thanked God for the freedom I felt entering my heart.

The fourth and fifth step bring inner peace, which heals anything. When this has been done thoroughly, you're ready for the sixth and seventh step — character defects.

Anger was my largest character defect. Now anger is a normal part of life, but not raging over *everything*. (Let me note here, it's imperative one be in the process of some mental clarity before attempting this step. Cerebral reactions are not a character defect — it's how we *act* on them that is.

Rage was my constant reaction to life's irritations. Unprovoked rage (out of nowhere — inappropriate) is also a byproduct of the yeast toxins on the hypothalamus. Whatever the reason is immaterial. To mend, I could not abuse others. When my cerebrals were out of control, as was I, I became violent with my children. The cerebral over, most of the time, I had no recollection of my behavior. Knowing this reaction is chemical is helpful in forgiving oneself. However, being human, I had to make amends in order to forgive myself completely.

Knowledge of the disease process is a strong tool in this forgiveness. Educating oneself thoroughly as to the physiologic and mental symptoms of the disease will alleviate the guilt associated with our actions during a reaction. Removing oneself from people to protect both of you also increases self-worth. Training friends and family to tell you when you're in a reaction is always heard by that inner spark, no matter how small. *We are not powerless.* We can master ourselves through these small steps. Finally, ask forgiveness for your behavior, whether chemical or emotionally induced. It doesn't matter how the other person responds. This is a selfish program to build up *your* self-worth. There are no half-measures. Amends improves self-esteem immensely.

When you're ready for the eighth and ninth step, you'll be amazed at how well you are getting. With sufficient clarity, you can begin making amends to anyone you've harmed. With the eighth step, I found myself at the top of the list. True forgiveness is a two-way street: first you must forgive *your* action or inaction, second you must forgive the unforgiveable. Remember this is for *you*.

Forgiving persons who had harmed me proved very tough. How could I forgive my mentally sick parents for all the damage done in childhood? Coming from an alcoholic home is a high-stress life. I'd learned to live life as a continual crisis. Combine this personality with genetic immune weaknesses, and you're set up for this type of breakdown.

Great tragedy had followed me throughout life: a brutal, abusive, poverty-stricken childhood, sexual molestation at age 4, rape age 22, a fatal attraction for verbally sadistic men, a disastrous marriage, crippled by my spine during divorce, the disease of alcoholism, and finally, candidiasis. How did I survive it all? Yes, I was a tough soul. *But E.I. floored me.* The barrel burst. No longer could I continue carrying this excess emotional baggage around with me and stay alive. It was that simple.

The amends steps saved my life. Within their simplicity, I found love and forgiveness. As I forgave myself, it became easier to forgive others. As I healed, I could clearly see people who'd harmed me were spiritually sick. They needed my forgiveness and blessings, not my hate. Sounds easy. *It wasn't. It still isn't.* My progress spiritually is a day at a time, with one step forward three backwards. The important part is to practice the steps daily to the best of one's ability. The disease spontaneously heals with each act of forgiveness. Grieving follows. For the E.I. sufferer like myself, it's important to let the tears flow. Crying heals. Love enters the body more and more with each healing. The spark of life grows and grows, til one notices one symptom after the other disappearing.

Yes, there is a long period of reconstruction. However, we should be sensible, tactful, considerate and humble without being servile or scraping. As God's people you stand on your feet; you don't crawl before anyone.

This thought brings us to Step 10. Each night before retiring (remember this is when you're able) ask yourself if you were resentful, angry, worried, dishonest or self-pitying. Forgive yourself. Now list the things you like that you did. I stayed alive. I was kind to an angry friend. I tried to follow the diet. Most importantly, give yourself credit for *trying*. For there are no failures, just lessons. From each mistake one can learn a new way. In the morning, ask the Creator that you be free of self-will and divorced from self-pity, anger, and self-seeking motives.

The eleventh step is prayer and meditation. Earlier, I mentioned another technique to deal with cerebrals. For those of you who pray, repeating over and over to yourself "behind the reaction" — just as if you were standing behind yourself — a rote prayer, or mantram, you will experience mastery of the cerebral. This simple technique can prevent suicide when you are alone, your therapist is not available, all your friends (if you have any left) have left town, and the hotline is busy. The rote repetition hypnotizes the subconscious and lessens the severity of the cerebral. Having self-mastery also adds to self-love. By doing this, I stopped myself from jumping out a window or running around wild in a maniacal reaction. Daily prayer of any kind heals. Pick some favorites. I've chosen the 23rd Psalm, and the St. Francis of Assissi Prayer:

> Lord make me an instrument of Thy peace. Where there is
> hatred, let me sow love; where there is injury, pardon; where

there is doubt, faith; where there is despair, hope; where there is darkness, light, and where there is sadness, joy.

O Divine Master, grant that I may not so much seek to be consoled as to console; to be understood as to understand; to be loved as to love. For it is in giving that we receive; it is in pardoning that we are pardoned, and it is in dying that we are born to eternal life.

For the more religious reader (those who can that is, read), the Book of Job will be very comforting in your despair and anger, while the Psalms seem to answer every need. Having never before read the Bible, I discovered a wonderful source of strength when mine ran out.

Meditation in any orthodox form is very difficult in the acute phases of this illness. I couldn't do it. But gentle forms exist. All you have to do is continue being collapsed on your bed. Take a deep breath to the count of 6 or as far as you can go. Hold it to the count of 6, then blow out every ounce of air, mentally releasing anger, rage, depression, bitterness, self-pity or fear. Repeat this as often as you can up to five minutes initially. A great deal of repair of the cells plus serenity, will begin from this humble exercise.

If you are strong enough, start visualizing a peaceful place you'd like to be. The beach or mountains is good for starters. Revel in this healing atmosphere. Only try five minutes til you're strong enough to build up to 15 minutes. Done several times daily, astounding recovery will result.

The most powerful meditation is one in which we contact the Source of All Energy. Hooking into this endless spring of healing energy can stop anaphylaxis, cerebrals, and vasculitis. Daily practice leads to a continuously strengthened channel. I was able to meditate when I was two years into recovery. Perhaps you will do it earlier or later. In any event, I can report the healing progressed in quantum leaps as my ability to meditate increased. Today, I meditate 15 to 20 minutes both morning and before retiring. If you'd told me this fact three years ago, I would have cynically said it was self-hypnosis. Well, it's a form of self-hypnosis, but on a higher level of consciousness. At the present time, I can pull myself out of a reaction, in which my left arm goes numb, with this advanced knowledge. My spiritual teacher is training me for my own healing ministry which is the culmination of my miraculous recovery from candidiasis.

Imaging is another powerful form of self-hypnosis or meditation. Meditation opened me up to a whole new world of healing which has presently evolved to very specific visualizations for the healing of candidiasis. Envisioning the specific body parts, then surrounding them with white or pink light engenders very rapid healing. I'll share a very special one with you.

The nervous system, the most severely damaged body part, needs the most help. Imagine a pink tree upside down, with its round root at the top. Physiologically, the nervous system resembles this image. Take three deep breaths, hold the third one for the count of twelve, and release your breath completely and fully. Sit quietly for five minutes initially, keeping the vision planted in your mind. Repeat to yourself, "My nervous system is the tree of life. I send pink healing light to all its branches I am healing. I am well." Try to build up to fifteen minutes gradually. But don't be discouraged if five minutes are difficult. Any attempt is a beginning. This particular image will heal the neurotoxic poisoning to the entire body.

Visualization techniques can be used on any organ in the body. They've been very successful with me. Perhaps this is the greatest tool for those of you who are physically unable to use anything orthodox medicine has to offer. Try it, you just might like it.

The twelfth step is helping others who suffer similarly to yourself. No matter how insignificant the help may seem to you, giving of oneself by sharing your experience, strength and hope will heal you. In fact, after self-love is initiated, service empowers the most intense healing of the body.

There is much more to these steps. By the time you've given these steps a thorough try, you'll notice a new awareness — self-acceptance.

When I accepted the fact that I had E.I., rather than fighting it or giving up in despair, recovery began. For healing cannot truly begin til we accept what *is* about ourselves. That's where mastery begins. My next step was to say, "Okay, this is what I have, I've chosen to live, now what do I do?" Losing that feeling of powerlessness channels new energy into the body, healing it. My experience proves that. I am functioning.

Eventually, I want to begin support groups to teach one another these powerful tools. In the meantime, Overeaters Anonymous uses the same steps and understands allergies. You don't have to be fat to join. Just desperate for support. They understand sugar cravings. In each city is a central office with names to call. Recovering foodaholics will help you by phone, if you will but ask. Several E.I.s have gone and been very grateful for the assistance. The totally isolated would gain phone contacts. *Many.* Depends on the size of your city or town. I've told E.I.s to explain that they are seriously ill and disabled in their homes. That's enough. For no one understands any further as they haven't lived it. So don't expect it.

I'd like to address the families of E.I.s briefly (if you still have one). At present, there is very little help for E.I.'s families who are confused, guilty and feel responsible to take care of you. The only solution I know of at present, and it's a good one, is to ask family members to attend Alanon or O-anon meetings in your area, the family auxiliaries of AA and OA. They will teach you how to detach from the sufferer's illness *with love*, without abandoning you or themselves in order to survive. I also highly recommend getting AA and OA's Big Book, replacing the word "alcohol" with "chemicals," and retaining OA's exact program.

Otherwise, be creative. Contact other families through E.I.A., HEAL, or CURE (formaldehyde poisoning) and form your own support groups. I guarantee you if you employ the knowledge presented here, your whole family will heal.

Reduce your expectations of yourself and others, particularly your family. Previously, I pronounced my high ideals to you. Ridiculously high expectations kept me in a state of high stress; high stress kept my muscles in a constant state of tension. Add to this the physical and mental tension brought on by candidiasis, plus the side effects of nystatin or Pau D'arco, from which muscle tension results, and you create a time bomb. Dealing with all this stress is enough. Now add to all this the idealistic personality and allergies to food, chemical and/or trees and weeds and you've produced a killer. One psychologist with E.I. told me that the "universal reactor" tended to be a super-survivor. I qualified. So do many E.I.'s I speak with by phone. The high stress came originally from unloving homes in childhood, whether it be alcoholic, or intellectually cold parents. Tons of high stress very early in life was a common thread among the critically ill.

Considering all these factors, we wind up with the highly intelligent, high energy, genetically allergic, "universal reactor" — most prone to the severest breakdown. I soon realized this described me. A change of attitude was the only solution. Employing the steps is one way of dealing with this attitudinal metamorphosis. In fact, for me, it's the only permanent way to growth. And spiritual growth results in emotional maturity. Emotional maturity produces freedom to live, explore, love and enjoy. Changing one's belief system, becoming non-judgmental just accepting what *is*, leads to the fullest enjoyment of life. But remember it's baby steps, a day at a time. My greatest challenge today is to be consciously aware of my negative thoughts or words and *change* them. This takes a lot of practice. It's a lot of fun and the results are prodigious. And guess what happens as a side effect of altering one's belief system? Candidiasis heals. I know — it happened to me.

Humor is another way to tap one's inner resources. Jokingly, I've told many people, if I jumped out a window in my suicidal cerebrals, I'd live, become a quadriplegic, and *still* have E.I. The way I see it, my time's not up yet. Nope.

Laughter pulled me through emotionally devastating moments. I shared my hilarious tale with many E.I.'s, for instance, about my first date, with oxygen when I was critically ill. Michael, a 36 year old auburn haired, bearded, six footer showed up. "Mind if I take my oxygen along?" "No," Michael said a little perplexed. In his van, my color turned yellow from the woodsmoke. When we arrived at the movie, I turned gray from the foggy rain. In the theater, I developed chest pain from the chemical smell. Losing consciousness began next. Tapping my date's arm, he accompanied me as I fell into the lobby. Laughingly he said, "Let's go from theater to theater and see how long we can last." I appreciated his wonderful sense of humor, but my person was blasted. So Michael suggested we go to his little house in the Oakland Hills. Half-dead, undaunted, I went. We sat on his couch, sharing ourselves. He gave me a glass of apple juice. Twenty minutes later, my entire body turned bright red, and I could see three of everything. Then the inevitable feeling of dying appeared. "Take me home, quickly!", I blurted as

I descended into shaking chills. He complied, very concerned. Back home, Michael bravely accompanied me to my 2nd floor bedroom. "Put me in bed, give me oxygen and cover me with every blanket you see. Please don't leave," I asked, trying to conceal my terror. "I won't." The reaction ended. Half-conscious, I raised my head saying "Isn't this the most unusual first date you've ever been on?" as I laughed heartily. "Yes," he said weakly.

Obviously, he rapidly dropped out of my life. But sharing this little vignette with fellow E.I.'s saved *my* integrity between the tears of rejection. Stubborn as I am, I tried anyway to date several more men while I existed in Berkeley. A 40ish, sexy, salt and pepper haired doctor tried to take me out. (I'd met him outdoors at Walnut Square, a chic woodsy shopping center in Berkeley on one of my better days.) Intelligent and witty, David seemed okay. Explaining E.I. to a biochemist-physician met with some understanding; blacking out in his marijuana-laced apartment didn't. On the patio, I tried for comfort: he wanted sex. Sex! Why if David had come any closer, he could be arrested for necrophilia!

In desperation for human contact, I hung out with fellow E.I.s. Joseph Mann and I survived by phone by regaling one another with stories of daily life with our common ailment. "Elizabeth, I went to the bank today. Five people were in line. By the time I reached the teller, I was ready to kill her." (Chemical reaction to perfume, hairspray etc. on people in line). I rolled on the floor laughing. Then I told him my tale. "Joseph, one day I went to San Francisco *before* I was completely isolated. A woman friend worried about leaving me alone in crime-swept Pershing Square. When she returned from Macy's, Nina queried.

"How did you do?"

"You should have seen it Nina. None of the weirdos or crazies bothered me. In fact, sitting here with my face covered by a carbon mask, they looked at me as if I were from outer space. *They* were afraid of *me*," I replied, cracking up.

Another even funnier event occurred last May. A visit with my chiropractor was absolutely hilarious. A healing crisis had placed my entire neck in spasm. Dr. Akers was accompanied by a chiropractic student.

"This lady has candidiasis. Last time she was here she looked like death warmed over."

"That was on one of my better days!" I announced, shaking the table with laughter.

We all enjoyed the irony of my situation.

When there were no outside sources of humor to tap (which frequently was the case), I ran tapes backwards in my head recreating *any* hilarious event in my past. There were many. Also, I'd laugh at the many bizarre ways I had to live. For example, whenever I went out with anyone, to attempt some connection to life, they had to get used to me dodging from spot to spot, avoiding cigarettes, paint fumes, diesel, and perfume. An outsider watching me would definitely call the white coats. Seeing the humor in our suffering is a powerful way to turn this tragedy into a healer. *Very powerful.* I laugh at *anything*. The more absurd the better.

As I was able to read and watch T.V. again, I read only comic books and stared at "Mash" addictively each night. These short spans of concentrated humor not only alleviated the stress, but healed my immune system. When I could go out, which was solo for a very long time, I took in funny movies or cartoons. The point being, surrounding oneself with humorous events lifts the spirit. It takes you out of yourself, even if its only for five minutes. In this way you give the body a break from the continual stress.

Walking is also very spiritual. Every day, I traipsed the Berkeley pier. The measure of time the walk took told me how sick or well I was. On good days, I could sprint the pier, both ways, in half an hour. On bad days, I'd almost crawl on all fours. Usually, an hour was sufficient. On toxic days, no walking was possible. Penetrating the mystique of the pier kept me busy. Fishing never before interested me. Yet I found myself talking to the various fishermen, learning about sea bass, mackerel and scrod, while hearing their philosophies on life. Amy would accompany me occasionally, looking with big dark brown eyes at the fishes' entrails being disemboweled. (Earlier she had begged me to take her fishing.)

"Mom, why do they do that to the poor fish?"

"They have to in order to prepare them for eating" came my sympathetic answer.

"Yuk, forget fishing! It makes me sick."

You never know who you'll meet on walks either. Surprisingly, someone loving and uplifting always appeared when I desperately needed it. Like Leo Bosco who I immortalized in my short story, "Another Encounter":

> The tall, lithe woman pulled into the parking lot next to the Bay and slipped her endless legs out the car door. Weak and faint, she decided to chance a walk along the pier and see if the fresh air would reverse her fatigue. The overcast sky showed peeks of sun, and a promise of total revelation before noon.

> Cautiously, she leaned on her car. The drug was reversing the illness, yet in turn, exhausting her at unpredictable moments. Praying for some time to walk and gain strength, she ambled slowly toward the path over the waters edge. All was well. Feeling stronger, she pulled her red fox jacket about her and allowed the cool March breezes to lash her face. How good it felt after three weeks on nystatin to be able to go for this walk and enjoy being out, without fearing perfume, mold or smoke; — the main agents that would cause her toxic body to collapse.

> How lucky she felt to be alive and able to enjoy this walk, no matter how short. Strength returned to her legs with each step forward and joy entered her heart. *I'm stronger, much stronger.*

> As she approached the pier whose phalanx pointed straight at the Golden Gate Bridge, she felt very shaky and couldn't

decide whether to go on or quit. After a brief talk to herself, she set out to walk the pier and watch the patient fishermen. Something made her turn back for a look at Berkeley. Approaching the pier, she spotted a tall well-dressed man coming her way.

Mmm, he looks interesting her mind's eye told her. How can I meet him without appearing too anxious? She did nothing and turned, then began her slow walk on the pier. She glanced back again. He was chatting with a fisherman at the pier's entrance. *Oh, well, he's not coming, so I'll go on.*

Feeling weak, she had to stop and lean on the mold covered guard rails. *O.K. go slowly, young woman, you've been seriously ill for six months.*

Again she began her trek, when the young stranger appeared right next to her. A fisherman was casting his reel and they both halted to let him.

The stranger turned and said, ''Is that a smelt?'' Shyly, she told him, ''I don't know. All fish look alike to me.'' She could smell the after-shave scent on him, and with trepidation, continued walking beside him. He didn't seem to mind. She took a good look and he pleased her. About 6'2'', very slim, sparkly hazel eyes, well tended medium brown hair, and an infectious personality. *A younger man would be fun for awhile.* Fantasies of him laughing and loving her danced in her brutalized brain.

Fantasies again. *I'm well, my brain is healing. Normal feelings are returning. This man is quite sexy.* He was visiting Berkeley for the day on business for handicapped people. A compassionate soul, she mused.

Rapidly, she blurted out the recovery from her illness, the severe isolation for the past six months from mankind. They chatted amicably until she felt weak. *Could be the after-shave.* She told him quietly, it was time to return to her car, as she was very weak. He came along and they sat on a worn wooden bench overlooking the Bay, and further discussed her closeness to her mortality and the profound change it wrought in her.

''I was a quasi jet-setter and that contributed to my downfall,'' offered Elizabeth. The man said, ''You must have given up a lot because of this.''

''Everything'' the woman replied.

He looked at her warmly and said ''You have a wonderful sense of humor.''

''Thank you,'' she declared. ''It's gotten me through life and now I feel great joy.''

At this point, his scent was weakening her badly and she jumped aside and said laughingly, ''Stay downwind, and I'll be safe.''

"O.K. By the way my name is Leo. What's yours?"
"Elizabeth, Elizabeth Rose."
"Leo Bosco."
"Really, as in the chocolate drink?"
'Yes," he laughed.

As they proceeded inland toward the boat moorings, he asked her plans for the future. She told him working with a biochemist who was also an inventor and had dispensed her to find a sharpie to manage his inventions. He knew how to do what she wanted. He gave her his card and they proceeded to a take-out food place in the Marina building, where she revealed she wrote and danced to gain equilibrium; playing piano and singing soothed him. Joyfully Elizabeth said "What a team we'd make!" Then he pulled back a bit.

Exhaustion set in, and Elizabeth beckoned him walk her back to the car. "I'll be here next Monday and I won't wear any scent. "Good," said she "we'll meet and see if you have what I'm looking for."

At the car he glanced at the toy in her back window.
"You have children?"
"Yes, two girls."
"Nice."
"How about you?"
"Yes, a daughter, 2 years old."
Embarassment, then silence.

He offered to follow Elizabeth to the freeway to be sure she was all right. She said yes. At the stop sign on University Avenue they waved goodbye forever.

The brief interlude with Leo brought kindness, compassion, and passion into my life for an hour — the most genuine concern from another human being I'd experienced physically in nearly six months.

Fantasy and walking were interchangeable for me. Whenever I met someone nice like Leo, I had something to take home inside of me. These precious jewels I cherished, calling on them again and again when times got rough. And there were many.

Gazing at San Francisco across the gray-green bay water and smelling the salty air, gave me visions of what I would do in that magical city when I became well. Go through the parks, speak to every bird on the grass, watch the tourists strolling, marveling at the city's beauty. The San Francisco Opera House, the art galleries, the cable cars. All would be mine again.

I'd look at every wave, search each plank of pier for splinters, graffiti and refuse. Each blade of grass in Berkeley Park had its own character. The seagulls chattered with one another. Kites flew in brilliant colors, painting the Berkeley skyline with stringed diamonds. Children played, running, falling, crying, squealing with joy. No one came very near me, but I went inside them without their even knowing it.

Walks brought new awareness of the neighborhood I lived in. Who lived in that house with the stained glass windows? A woman age 37, green-eyed frosted blonde hair. Loving, but uptight, with her lawyer husband. Two children. Both boys. The four year old blond and whining; the eight year old a miniature adult with eyeglasses. Look at that man lovingly watering his roses. The blue eyes soft and knowing, the hands surviving many thorns. All made up of course, but it fills the long lonely hours.

The fantasy is endless walking. Seeing a tree, leaf by leaf, shaped as a sweeping splendor. Learning of flowers, petal by petal. And let me not leave out how marvelously invigorating fresh air is when your head is fogged or you are nauseated; the walk clears it. As I walk, I inhale to the count of twelve, hold it til six, release it to the count of six. By repeating this twelve times, you aerate the entire system. Kriya Yoga lessons taught me these techniques. Combining walking with breathing techniques has a very peaceful effect. Harmony fills the mind. No matter how small the perambulating, the movement moves toxins out of the body.

Which brings me to singing and dancing as a healing aid. Dancing was an avocation I'd enjoyed most of my life,— til candidiasis. Dancing represented a form of transcending every day life. Losing it almost squelched my spirit. Joseph would come to visit me in Berkeley. With the lights on 25 watt, I'd create a ballet scene. Thinking myself stronger than I was, I'd get carried away, dance passionately for five minutes, then fall on the couch gasping for breath. It didn't matter — we had fun and it fortified my direction emotionally — I was healing.

Singing funny songs helped too. The more raunchy the better. My girls and I would sing naughty songs and crack up laughing. Naughtiness is cultivated in my home. For it's the child in me at play, and my ability to play which saved my life.

Play takes many forms. I literally ''played'' with Jean-Pierre a great deal of the time. Creating fantasies about my attempts to go out, alleviated the trauma from what actually happened. We'd pretend we were children running away from home on an adventure through our own neighborhood. We'd run (short ones) and hide behind the trees. Jean-Pierre couldn't find me. Bump, I'd appear, kiss him gently on the neck. Or we'd pretend we were in Paris, viewing the wonderful art. So what if I fell out the door of the studio in real life. The important point was — I did it at all.

When I moved back to Santa Monica a brain scientist friend at UCLA hearing of my dilemma, told me that healing for candidiasis was spiritual, and drawing stimulated right brain functioning — the creative center. Drawing! In high school, I'd given that up when intimidated by the natural born artists in my class. Today, I am drawing somewhat, mainly visions or scenes

I experience in dreams. It's soothing. Seems I'd been doing all right brain activity intuitively right along to heal myself. Agnes verified what I already knew: that the healing comes from within using one's own inner resources.

Dreams became very instrumental in my later recovery, as I learned to work with their powerful messages. Brenda taught me to start a daily dream diary, whereby I kept a pencil and notebook at my bedside and jotted down the dreams half-asleep, as they occurred.

Whenever fears of chemicals or foods showed up, I surrendered on bended knee, (or lying down) the fears to God upon awakening: the reaction to that particular substance would disappear within days. Incidents from the past would resurrect, childhood for instance, in which I experienced long forgotten scars. By visualizing the negative image of myself in conscious awareness, and going into that dream in a meditative state, I'd talk to the frightened girl lovingly, offering her God's light, love and compassion. Within days, I'd feel lighter and the imaging would spontaneously heal my body further! Presently, I'm planning to teach a seminar on this particular type of healing, for it has extremely rapid results.

But what about me you say, who can't dance, draw, write, jump, laugh, or dream anymore? What about me who is so debilitated I can't read, use a pen or pencil, watch T.V., listen to tapes or records. What about me? Who can't be touched, who's dying of loneliness and isolation. I've been there. This last entry is for you.

When I was that ill, and hopeless despair was my constant companion, everyone and everything failed me. I couldn't live. Only exist. Jean-Pierre, too far away to comfort me physically; my old friends were far away at the other end of the state. When I couldn't face another minute of my torture chamber body; when I didn't want to live another minute, even for my children; when I couldn't bear the pain of the loneliness and isolation for one more second — I did two things.

First, I'd lie half-alive, on my bed or couch. Then I'd run the tape of my life before my eyes. Over and over, I re-ran the good things: the successes, the joys, the heights, the funny events, the loving events. Sometimes I'd project into the future. Fantasies of visiting Europe. Greece in particular. I'd plan the entire trip in my mind. Or I'd make plans for what career I'd choose when I became well. *Writing a book of my story. Writing articles. Planning meeting publishers in my head. Where I'd live. What schools to send my girls to best nurture them.* Pleasant thoughts. Loving thoughts. Healing thoughts. Better times were coming.

Until they did, my second tool worked under any circumstances. This "crutch" was my saviour when I was in anaphylaxis, vasculitis attacks, close to dying, terrified, in cerebrals, all together or separately, and felt totally abandoned by life and wanted life to abandon me.

I'd lay on my bed (or floor) and scream out to the Creator "Heal me or take me." A flow of warmth would flood my body. Whatever circumstance was threatening my life or sanity, it stopped. Let me share here the first time this happened to me, in October of '81, during the three weeks of anaphylactic shock. Not quite believing in a Supreme Being, and writhing in agony on my bed from my heart pounding at around 200 beats a minute, while my skin glowed bright red and burned, and the sensation of dying permeated my being, I cried out for my dead mother. ''Mama help me, help me,'' I begged, tears streaming down my face, which rapidly changed to, ''If there is a God,help me!''

Without warning, a deluge of warmth flooded my entire body. Everything became motionless, timeless. The room felt unreal, as if I were not a part of the world. I was bathed in a rocking, fluidish feeling sensation which I can only describe as bliss. An unparalleled feeling of joy or bliss, way beyond what one could ever experience on earth. I was given a choice to stay with God or come back. I wanted to stay with Him, in this state, eternally. He then told me it wasn't my time — I had to go back. I didn't want to return. He said I must. I didn't understand, but agreed.

The room became natural again. A quiet peace filled my being. Puzzled and awestricken, I had no idea what had happened to me. The acute continuous anaphylactic reactions of the past three weeks and all other symptoms stopped for awhile. Never again did I return to such a *concentrated* state of near death. Yet, there were many times after that, between 30 and 50 times (I didn't keep count — too ill) over the next 2½ years where I faced death again. At these critical times, I employed another avenue to God. For, most important of all, when it took all my strength to whimper ''Help me'' or I was only semi-conscious and I couldn't ask for help, *some "force" took care of me.* For earlier in my illness, I'd surrendered my life and will to God.

And finally, when you're in cerebrals, and there is no God, and there is complete separation from self and you want to commit suicide, a spark exists to which we are attached and our despair is felt. *We are always watched and cared for.* In our sane moments, *we have to ask for help to be protected in our toxic episodes.* It's that simple. *We have to ask for help.* That's all there is. And God is everything. He will not abandon you. He will never let you down. *Never.*

BLESSINGS AND LESSONS

Could I conclude this book without enumerating the blessings that have entered my life as a result of my multiple brushes with death? I think not. For without perceiving my trial by fire as a baptism, I'd have entirely missed the point, and be doomed to repeat the past. The thought of living through this experience one more time is more than I can bear. Therefore, I'll share the sunshine that came into my life..

I learned I wasn't infallible, that high stress and genetic weaknesses exact a price.

. . . I was worthwhile dying, not being a perfect mother, not earning a living, not producing. Just being.

. . . who I really was — a talented dynamo with a weakness for pathological men.

. . . to let go of being overresponsible, thereby attracting parasitical people to drain me. (I'm still at this one.)

. . . that God takes care of children when I can't. All I have to do is ask Him.

. . . that children have emotional scars despite a parent's best intentions — they do have their own personalities.

. . . to reach out and ask for help, which I previously couldn't do. This resulted in learning a healthy dependence on people, which blossomed into healthy independence.

. . . I didn't have to be with abusive men because I was ill, that I was totally loveable, no matter what my physical condition.

. . . that the physical body is not important, the inner spirit is what really counts. This helped me to accept myself emaciated and gray, fat and bloated from nystatin.

. . . I deserve love just for being me.

. . . there is a "force," whom I choose to call God, who has left me awestricken with his love and mercy for me.

. . . to stop beating myself up mentally and praise my efforts.

. . . to hug myself and when I couldn't let the Lord do it.

. . . to love myself. No one can take that from me.

. . . life is a daily progression — there are no mistakes, just lessons.

. . . trusting a Higher Power brought me everything I needed not only to survive, but live fully.

. . . to trust myself.

. . . to feel my feelings, and let them go. Previously, I fought, denied, or ignored them.

. . . by becoming a loving person I attracted loving people.

. . . there are many decent people in the world, who will love and help you as best they can.

. . . to accept myself as less than perfect as having physical limitations.

. . . more thoroughly to see the challenge in my personal tragedy rather than succumbing to self-pity.

. . . to take til I reached a balance where I could give and take.

. . . my children developed a source of faith that sustained them through this incredibly lengthy crisis.

. . . I used all my resources for the first time in my life to heal myself.

. . . you can heal from any degenerative disease if you choose to live.

. . . there's a Divine Plan, which I far from know its entirety, in which the Maker sometimes chooses us to live for a reason.

. . . that illness is not bad, just *is*, a gift and a lesson.

. . . that life exists after death and it's more beautiful than anyone can imagine.

. . . that hard times bring good friends.

. . . that the Creator is the only one we can depend on totally in the whole universe.

. . . that inner peace is everything.

. . . that life can be enjoyed seriously ill.

. . . that learning to love oneself is tough but an endlessly rewarding journey.

. . . that the death of the ego is the beginning of life.

. . . that disease is an opportunity to learn to love yourself, which I missed doing as a child.

. . . a disease can be a protection in childhood from trauma.

I believed the human spirit was indomitable and I proved it.

. . . that we could choose to live or die. My journey reaffirms this belief.

. . . love can heal anything. It did.

I discovered inner resources and talents I didn't know I had, thereby opening up a whole new world for me.

. . . my true reason for living — to love, employing all my talents and inner essence.

. . . hatred and bitterness enervate the body, therefore weakening the immune system.

. . . the reason for surviving was to help the others behind me.

. . . I healed from childhood abuse, opening my heart to love through an innocent child's eyes.

But most of all, I acquired the knowledge that love is what life is all about. Today I'm surrounded with it: in my work, my children, my friends, my home, my business acquaintances. When I see the absence of love, I send blessings to that poor, unloved soul (not perfect at this folks) and move on. Negative people aren't in my life today. That is a transformation.

For Environmental Illness humbled me, reducing my status to that of a small dependent child, which forced me to change or perish. It was through this devastating lesson that I let go of the pseudo-adult in me and re-discovered the curious, vulnerable, risking, fun-loving, laughing child. A playful, awe-stricken child — full of curiosity about life.

And so I became truly alive for the first time in my life, echoing the words of Christ uttered nearly 2000 years ago:

". . . unless you change and become like little children, you
will not enter the kingdom of God. (Matthew 18:3).''

And so I recaptured the wonder of living all over again, through the eyes of an innocent child.

OTHER ALTERNATIVE THERAPIES

A deluge of questions about alternative therapies led me to share my experiences with other modalities:

1) Acidophilus — Whether from milk or non-dairy forms, lactobacillus acidophilus was not tolerated by my body. During the acute stage I tried a tiny amount and experienced no changes in my condition. A non-dairy powder I tested recently produced severe reactions manifested as toxic bloat and weight gain, continuous food cravings, constipation, cement-like abdomen, bleeding swollen gums with fever blisters on my palate, and severe brain fog, anxiety and obsessive thinking — and I am symptom free of Candida. I had milk allergy at birth coming close to dying. My reaction demonstrates what milk does to lactose sugar-sensitive peoples' bodies imperceptibly over the years. The non-sensitive sufferers claim acidophilus is very beneficial. A carrot-dophilus for the lactose-sensitive can be obtained through Dr. Stephen Levine. A new product, that kills Candida, taurine-acidophilus developed by Hanna Kroeger, is having amazing results.

2) Acupuncture — It's wonderful! It builds up the immune system and balances the body's energy so it can heal itself. Whenever I binge on sugar, I contact Dr. Luc for a treatment. In my critical phase of Candidiasis, anaphylaxis sometimes resulted from acupressure. So I'd proceed slowly with acupuncture.

3) Bifidus — The smell nauseated me. Again not for the lactose-sensitive.

4) Caprylic Acid — A fatty acid from a coconut base. Caprystatin made me ill, faint and my abdomen blew up to balloon size on one pill. I feel it is stronger than nystatin and must be used just as carefully. If you are coconut sensitive this may not be for you. Capricin and Dr. Stephen Levine's Caprylate Plus are getting great results in some patients. Dr. Levine's is especially beneficial due to the balance of L-Taurine and other key nutrients in his product. It is one of the essential amino acids responsible for cell mediated-immunity which is either missing, destroyed or not formed in Candidiasis.

5) Chiropractors — Excellent. In the later stages of recovery after a

healing crisis I found my back and neck went out. An adjustment released the muscle spasm and toxins trapped in the tissues. As always I proceeded slowly so as not to enter a ferocious detox.

6) Colonics — I found they depleted my strength far too much in the critical phase of the illness. As I became much stronger, a warm water modified home colonic (I used an enema bag, laid on my left side, filled the colon till the slightest discomfort, evacuated the water, laid on my back lifting my hips repeating the procedure, then laid on my right side and completed the same). My head cleared and toxic gases from die-off that would have been reabsorbed into my system were eliminated. I waited at least three days between colonics so as not to exhaust myself. I really believe my healing accelerated by preventing the toxic wastes from being recirculated. I continue to do them occasionally as a cleansing, especially after a Haagen-Daz or croissant episode.

7) Homeopathic Remedies — Due to my intolerance for lactose, sugar and alcohol I could not use them as they are usually preserved in these substances. They do help people who do not have these limitations.

8) Massage — Great! Not only does it feel good (you get touched) it releases toxins and facilitates healing. I went slowly on this as it can induce a healing crisis.

9) Mercury-amalgam filling removal — Mention dental work and I freak! A new non-petrochemical based binder exists but I haven't found it yet. I find filling-removal extreme but hear it helped some people but is not a cure while others got sicker from the new materials. The body goes through a detox with each amalgam removal so again I'd progress slowly, one a month or so. My gumline cavity began remineralizing and the decay arrested as a result of using the KIVA light. In any case if I don't know what to do I go within and seek my own inner guidance.

10) Ozone therapy — My body reacted so negatively on ionizers which produce ozone I decided an invasive procedure would be dangerous. The less sick cases are helped in some instances however.

11) Trampoline — This little gadget is marvelous for clearing your head. I was able to use it as I became stronger and mobile. It cleanses the malfunctioning lymph system. Try it — you'll have fun.

The two biggest questions I'm asked over and over are: Is this contagious? do we have AIDS? NO! NO! to both. If it were contagious my two daughters would be critically ill or dead. My experience shows me that only an already depressed immune system in an individual would bring on this breakdown. Candida is an opportunistic host meaning the body must be under serious environmental and emotional stress for this to occur. It *is* acquired immune deficiency as are all auto-immune disorders but our path is quasi-allergic reactions whereas AIDS victims develop Kaposi's sarcoma and a deadly form of pneumonia along with systemic Candida. I believe the overgrowth of Candida, an organism found naturally in the body is the end product, not the cause, of life out of balance.

AFTERWORD

As many of you know, this book is ahead of its time, and remains so, with the result my readers' curiosity builds: What happened after you published LADY OF GRAY in 1985. In fact, the most oft asked questions are: How are you doing *now?*; Are your reactions gone?; Can you lead a normal life? Did you marry Tom?; What effect did this have on your children?; Are you *really* well?

One by one, I will answer your questions only for the purpose of allaying your fears that there is little or no hope of *permanent* recovery. But first I must clarify one thing. People with Candida, untreated and unhealed, *usually,* but not always, evolve into Environmental Illness which is not a separate disease but the final stage of systemic Candidiasis. This physical breakdown is not "allergy" but toxic poisoning. Therefore if you have a "touch" of Candida and someone promises you an instant "cure", beware. In the advanced stages, excluding a miracle from God, this condition takes years to turn around, a slow and painful process at best, yet immensely rewarding in the end, for the joys and blessings will amaze you. Each of you who do make it through, patiently utilizing the knowledge in this book, will find yourselves in a different state of mind and a different way of living. Talents you never dreamed you possessed will emerge. Being an entrepeneur working from your home is the vision I see. Others will turn to helping people in some productive way, enhancing society. And those of you who are presently critically ill—you are the Light in your city, the example. Your very survival and recovery will be the only job you need accomplish to show the world God's purpose in all this horror, this purpose being to hang on to God's coattails for answers in a way previously unknown to you as you journey back to a spiritually centered being.

As for me, I am totally free of reactions unless exposed to freshly sprayed pesticides, paint or varnishes *in sealed buildings.* I then remove myself rapidly from the environment, my left arm goes slightly numb, and within minutes I'm fine again. Those unfortunate souls sitting in these toxic workplaces have no idea what they are being exposed to and what can happen to them. Well-ventilated, non-toxic buildings are being built by "the awake". Keeping a safe home [mine is a normal disaster area, but remains chemically free of the major polluters] provides a mental sanctuary. If this sounds down, remember thousands are joining us each day and we, the pioneers, are the new leaders who will have to turn around this toxic planet.

Having had anaphylaxis too many time too count, it was the last symptom to leave. The KIVA Light continues to heal my adrenals, my body now reacting only on poisons placed directly in my body, like dental glue—I have found the non-toxic replacement—and I continue to find many safe alternatives to chemical usage in my home.

Healing crises continued to appear from time to time, however, I was fully functioning energy-wise long before my body had completed its healing from old damage, writing book after book, sit-coms and screenplays, working on breaking into the movie industry, my next-door neighbor here, and finding a producer to to make a film of my [our] story.

The hardest part of my recovery has been emotionally, returning to life extremely gradually after being so violently ill and isolated for so many years. The

12 Steps I mentioned in the text helped me through this very difficult period and I continue using them for everything imaginable that comes up in daily life. After learning patience, you learn more patience.

Tom committed suicide in March of '88. Never quite beleiving that I knew anything, he didn't use the tools I employed and deteriorated rapidly in 1987. It took me a long time to recover from that tragedy though Tom had drifted out of my life the two years prior. Not everyone makes it. Our destiny is truly in God's mind.

I'd be a liar if I told you my children came through this horror unscathed. Nevertheless, this adversity brought out the strengths in both of them, Amy pursuing a musical and acting career, Jen blossoming more and more in her artistic talent as she attends college.

But am I really well? Let's say I look at recovery from E.I. the same way I deal with my recovering from alcoholism. A day at a time, I am well in that moment. That's all any of us have anyway. That thinking keeps me healthy. High energy flows from me nearly continuously except when I hit a healing crisis—they do change in intensity and eventually become like a bad cold—deep cleansing my body at another level, always leaving me stronger, healthier and extremely creative. I credit the KIVA Light and my spiritual program with the permanent healing and lack of reversals to my prior state, no matter what hits me.

Still have all my teeth, still fear going to *any* dentist—the KIVA light keeps my mouth in good shape—still find removing mercury unnecesary. Heal the immune system first, the body stops reacting on all chemicals. That is still my experience.

The best hope I can share in my eighth year of making it is you will be symptom free one day and not have to live the bizarre existence we are forced into. It's a long haul, truly depending on how sick you were to begin with. But you are functioning well long before the body has completed its healing. After the healing is completed you must continue to guard against breaking the body down again.

If I can have my roof repaired by environmentally alert roofers without having to move out or becoming seriously ill, that should answer any question of how well I am.

Nothing new under the sun has surfaced regarding the healing of this illness since I wrote the book in 1984, just new twists on alternative therapies. They all work, and one must find what suits them best.

The planet is undergoing a revolution, forcing mankind to turn back to a sane way of living. The planet's hope in this polluted era lies in you and your family hearing God's wonderful creation cry out "Stop! We need to undo what we have done." The solution begins with you in any small way. Each step forward in your own recovery heals the planet. I pray I have helped you to heal.

(Elizabeth Rose has been honored in *Who's Who In American Women 1989-90* and *THE INTERNATIONAL BIOGRAPHERS OF WORLD LEADERS 1990-91,* Cambridge, England, for her contributions to assisting the world with her knowledge of chemical poisoning and its reversal.)

CANDIDA DIET

1. Proteins — steamed or baked
   Chicken, fish, beef, turkey, duck, eggs, seafood, goat, venison, rabbit, quail and lamb. Essentially all meats, *chemically free* if available in your area. No dried, smoked, pickled or cured meats.

2. Starches — steamed corn, rice, millet and potatoes in small amounts.

3. Vegetables — all vegetables are fine. Sweet potatoes and potatoes may have to be avoided temporarily. *No raw.*

4. Liquids — Plenty of bottled water. Fresh comfrey is okay for tea. Otherwise, no teas.

5. *No* fruits, fruit juices, commercially prepared foods, condiments, sugar, honey, dairy products or grains except as previously mentioned.

6. Vitamins and minerals — Most products contain yeast and chemicals. Check labels for ingredients.

7. Oils — fresh olive oil and some vegetable oils can be tolerated. Water and oil or lemon and oil make a tasty dressing.

8. Butter — tolerable if no chemicals (raw) and melted down in a pan with the curds and cream skimmed off.

The diet is temporary. Remember that thought. Following it will remove stress from your body, enabling it to begin healing itself.

FOR INDIVIDUAL CONSULTATION
WITH ELIZABETH ROSE
PHONE
(213) 829-2002

ORDER FORM

(ORIGINAL FORM MUST ACCOMPANY
YOUR ORDER FOR DISCOUNT)

Interested in further information as to *how* I accomplished the inner healing of systemic Candidiasis and how I *stay* well?

Yes, I would like the following tapes: (Mark X beside tapes you wish to order)

_____1. 12 SPIRITUAL STEPS OF RECOVERY: A beginner's $ 9.95
introduction to forgiveness and letting go of resentments based on AA's 12 steps

_____2. VISUALIZATIONS FOR THE PHYSICAL HEALING: $ 9.95
Enlightened guided imagery for specific body parts affected by Candidiasis

_____3. COMFORTING AFFIRMATIONS AND $ 9.95
MEDITATIONS TO LESSEN REACTIONS: An excellent tape to heal fear and not feel alone during reactions.

_____4. OPTIMUM USE OF INNER RESOURCES TO $ 9.95
MAINTAIN YOUR INTEGRITY AS A HUMAN BEING: Practical everyday reminders to keep yourself calm, centered and relaxed and not lose friends and family.

Add $2.00 for shipping and handling per tape
or ALL 4 tapes — $6.00

Do you need an extra copy of *Lady of Gray* for a friend?   _____ Yes
Special Price with this order form - $13.00 plus $2.00 shipping

BUTTERFLY PUBLISHING COMPANY
2210 Wilshire Blvd.
Suite 845
Santa Monica, Calif 90403

Include your

Name ______________________________   Tel No. ______________________

Address ____

City __________________________   State ______________   Zip __________